D1564680

The Year THEY Tried to Kill Me:

Surviving a surgical internship… even if the patients don't

Salvatore Iaquinta, MD

Purely Chaotic Publishing

Copyright © 2012 Salvatore Iaquinta

All rights reserved.

Version 4.1 – now with invisible typos!

ISBN: 0988434911

ISBN-13: 978-0-9884349-1-2

To everyone who helps me become better.

Disclaimer

Everything I wrote was my perception of reality at the time I wrote it. Some people might argue certain events happened differently. Those people can write their own books. Names of people, sex, race, and even eye color have been altered to protect the innocent and guilty alike.

Laughter is the best medicine, but surgery is a close second.

CONTENTS

Preface

If you are a fourteen-year-old boy, you probably cannot imagine anything worse than going to the doctor's office and getting a rectal exam.

And if Joshua knew that his complaint would lead to such an invasion of privacy, I am sure he wouldn't have told his mom that he had a burning sensation at the tip of his penis after urinating.

I met Joshua and his mother first, while my attending physician saw another patient. Joshua wore a sweatshirt advertising the Green Bay Packers, blue jeans, and basketball shoes. His mom looked like every teenager's mom, putting on a little weight and a lot of concern.

The fact that Josh had his mom with him in the room revealed his naiveté. Any sexually active young man who knows of the existence of STDs would have banished his mother from the examination room before any discussion began. But Josh didn't hesitate to describe the short-lived stinging feeling in his penis after urinating; therefore, he wasn't sexually active.

He needed a full genital and rectal exam. I decided to be polite and wait for the attending physician so we could perform the exam together. I pointed to the folded gown on the examination table. "Why don't you put that on so we can examine you while I escort your mom to the waiting room?"

I ditched mom in the overcrowded lobby, found Dr. Bissle, and presented Josh's case. "Well, what do you think it is?" he asked. He always kept a perfect poker face during a presentation, as if every piece of information was equally unimportant.

"He could have a urinary tract infection or he could have an STD if he were lying about sexual activity," I said. "Of course, at this age, lying about sexual activity would more likely be a lie in favor of having sex, not one of abstinence." I paused for Dr. Bissle to acknowledge my witticism, but it didn't happen.

"Or, he could have prostatitis, which can cause burning at the end of urination. That means we should do a rectal." Notice I said we. I meant him. If I did the rectal, he would have to do it again to verify my findings. I disapprove of redundant rectal intrusion, unless someone really deserves it.

Dr. Bissle rapped on the door twice and quickly opened it. Joshua sat on the table in his gown, scratching at a pimple on his jaw. Dr. Bissle watched me examine Joshua's lower abdomen and genitals before giving him the bad news. "Joshua, I am going to have to do a rectal exam. If your prostate is inflamed, it can cause your symptoms."

Joshua went white. I read his mind. That burning isn't so bad, why did I tell my mom about it? I'll never discuss my health with that backstabber again!

Dr. Bissle grabbed a pair of Latex gloves from the wall. "You will feel like you need to go to the bathroom, but you won't." I watched him snap the gloves over his hands, which were easily one glove size smaller than mine. Lucky for Josh.

Joshua didn't hear him. I imagined he was preoccupied with thoughts of what his friends would say if they found out.

Dr. Bissle squeezed some surgical lubricant on his finger. The frightened young man curled up on his side like a little boy, and he winced as Dr. Bissle inserted his finger and massaged his prostate. If he had prostatitis, he would have flown across the room.

I saw a wave of relief pass across Josh's face as the Dr. Bissle removed his finger. I grabbed a tissue and handed it to him.

"Thanks," he said softly as he took the tissue and used it to wipe away a tear.

I bit my cheek and quickly grabbed another tissue. "Here, you can wipe away the extra lubricant."

The boy looked at me with an air of understanding.

Doctor Bissle explained to Joshua that his prostate exam was normal. We went out into the hallway to give him a chance to dress before talking to him and his mother.

As soon as we got out of earshot I burst out laughing. Dr. Bissle looked at me quizzically, undoubtedly wondering if I got my giggles by watching teenage boys get rectal exams. I told him about the tissue. He actually smiled.

Now, I know what you are thinking. How can they let such an immature person become a doctor?

I ask myself that every day.

Chapter 1

Thirteen of us sat around a conference table, waiting for the chief resident to arrive. It was seven-thirty in the morning, probably earlier than any of us had woken up in the few weeks since medical school ended. But coffee was unnecessary; every one of us brimmed with nervous energy.

Dr. Organ, the chairman of the surgical program, came in first, to say good morning. He contemplated the chair at the head of the table as if he wasn't sure we were worth the effort to sit down and stand back up for the few moments he'd spend with us. But then he sat.

He took a second to look right through each of us. His crisp white coat contrasted his black skin. He sat with a perfect posture that hinted of military training or a very strict mother. We all unconsciously sat up straight in our chairs, already under his command.

But once he started talking, he seemed like a cheerful grandfather figure: gray hair, witty jokes, and a big smile. He was probably a pleasure to work with. We believed his sound bites. *Everything will be great if you work hard. Everything will be great if you work enthusiastically. This will be one of the most exciting years of your life.*

By the time Dr. Organ stood up to leave, we had all relaxed in our chairs. As he exited, I noticed he walked with a limp. Despite his charming intro, I could imagine only one reason why he'd have a limp. He probably got an arthritic hip from years of kicking interns. That's what chairmen do.

Then, the chief resident entered and sat at the head of the table. He looked at us, the new interns, and smiled—the kind of smile a cat gives a mouse. He wasn't nearly as tall as Dr. Organ, nor as impressive in appearance. Short, skinny white guys just like him infested the medical field, the kind of guys that argued with the teacher from the third grade on. Nonetheless, he earned the title chief resident, one of four in charge of all the residents and interns at Highland Hospital.

He was close enough to us in age that no one stiffened up in his or her chair as he sat down. He, too, had perfect posture. As for me, I sat slouched in my chair. I clearly didn't have military training or a strict mother. Maybe my posture would improve while I was there; my mom would be happy.

"Good morning everyone, I am Dr. Bradford, one of the chiefs. Does anyone have any questions before I begin?"

"Yes," I asked. "What book should we be reading this year?" I needed the User's Guide to the Surgical Internship, if such a book existed.

"I'll get to that later. Any other questions?"

All right, I'm patient.

"How is call organized?" One of the interns asked. He looked like he just finished night call, tired and unshaven. And he had those wrinkles at the corner of his smile that you don't get until you breach forty. There was something shady about him. Shady Man.

"I'll get to that later," Dr. Bradford answered.

Someone else asked a question. Dr. Bradford told us he would get to it later.

"Any others?" Dr. Bradford waited 1.2 seconds, during which no one bothered to ask about dictation, operating procedure, expectations, clinic, conferences, locker rooms, call rooms, or dress code. "Well, if there are no more questions, I will get started. Feel free to ask any that might pop into your head."

I smiled, but nobody else found this amusing.

"Who here doesn't own the new Palm 5x?" he asked. As his eyes took a lap around the conference table, no one moved. We looked like stereotypic twenty-somethings: khakis (not on me), button-down shirts, a few wedding rings, but not on any of the five women. Slacks and shirts for them, too; no dresses. We didn't look like doctors. The chief had a white coat, but the rest of us looked like we could be sitting in the college commons. No, worse. We looked like the group from the office going to TGI Friday's for lunch.

I wondered if they were afraid, or if they all had Palm Pilots? I didn't own one. Was it required? The looks on the others' faces told me they thought the same. I meekly raised a hand. The older-looking guy, Shady Man, maintained eye contact and slowly raised his hand, too. Ahh, safety in numbers. For that moment we were best friends.

The chief looked disappointed. "It isn't required. But it makes life easier. I do everything on this." He proceeded to pull his Palm Pilot from his pocket and demonstrate all of its marvelous functions. He even had scanned anatomy pictures into it. I wondered if my immediate disdain toward the little gadget would wane and I would succumb to buying one. Were there more reasons to hate it than it just being yuppie nerd gear? Probably, but I couldn't think of any. Wait, surgeons don't look at pictures while operating; shouldn't that information be in their heads? Especially his head—it was so big. Maybe his glasses were too small. No, his forehead was big and gleaming. Plenty of room for a billboard: Buy the Palm 5x!

After he had won over the crowd with his amazing Palm Pilot, he stressed the importance of organization ad nauseam. "An intern's only job is to know the patients better than everyone else. Information on a patient is finite, so you can know it all. You want the chief's trust. A chief can trust a knowledgeable intern," he said. The speech lost its threatening edge when he made it into a bribe. I want to be trusted! Me, me, me!

He paused and looked down at his Palm Pilot. He scrolled through his speech outline. Nerd gear.

"The one thing they can't do is stop the clock," he read.

Some people looked puzzled, including me.

"No matter what they do to you, they cannot stop the clock. It is only twelve months, and you get one of them off. Always remember that this is only one year of your life," Dr. Bradford said. He looked at each one of us like a teacher delivering a lecture. "Some people will be absolutely rude to you. Some surgeons will degrade you; some will grill you. Sometime near the beginning a nurse will call you up at two in the morning to ask you to renew a Tylenol order. Always remember that they are just fucking with you. Renew the order and go back to sleep. If you try to fight it, it will only happen more often. If you do what they want, they will stop.

"If a surgeon tries to break you, don't. Remember that they are trying to break you. Let their insults roll off you like a bead of water. If you snap back once, it will haunt you. Nobody here forgets anything. You will be paid back every day if you bite once. Do not cry. Even at home, do not cry. Remind yourself that it is only one year and that you just got through one more day. I have seen some great people leave this program because they couldn't take it. I've been to the East Coast and this is much worse. They are ruthless here," Bradford said without a smile. He delivered this information with the same flat affect he would use to describe a patient's vitals. These weren't opinions, these were the facts.

Nobody smiled. Our rosy expectations of starting our surgical training were replaced by the cold fact that we were now prisoners. At least our guy on the inside took the time to tell us how to deal with the guards.

I had avoided the East Coast because of the horror stories. The difference between the East and West Coast's training programs was that in the East they stab you in the back, whereas in the West you will see it coming. At the time, I thought that would mean the West wouldn't be so bad. But now I was scared; I'm a Midwest softy. I wanted my mom. There's no place like home, there's no place like home.

Maybe he was just trying to start the breaking. He wanted to see if someone would bolt. I looked around the table. Everyone looked as unexcited as a zombie, but no one scrambled for the door.

"I am telling you this so that you expect the worst. If you expect the worst, your experience might be better than you expect." Bradford raised his eyebrows as encouragement. "Give it a week. Everything happens in a week around here. You need a week to see what the clinics, conferences, and operating room schedules are like."

His sales pitch sucked. Why'd I sign up for this?

"Take a look around. Half of you won't be here four years from now. The attrition rate here is incredible. They don't really kick people out of the program; it's more like people disappear. But, if you do poorly on your yearly exams, and you aren't a good clinician, they might not renew your contract."

He proceeded to stress the importance of being liked by the staff, especially Dr. Organ. Being liked would make things easier. I might be one of the people allowed to do a year of research if he liked me. Being considered lucky to have a year off to do research shows how lousy this program is. Why else would a surgeon-in-training take a year off from operating to sit in a stinky lab dissecting rats, analyzing blood, or running gene sequences? I'd rather do rectal exams ungloved than research.

Dr. Organ didn't seem like an ogre. He didn't intimidate us; he smiled too much. Maybe he smiled at the thought of fresh meat. His limp really was from kicking residents' butts! The more Dr. Bradford talked, the more my image of Dr. Organ changed. Dr. Organ will ceaselessly question us on minutia. He will yell at us. He will be insulted if our pager goes off during a conference, so we had better set it on vibrate. If we get a page from his office we answer it immediately, no matter what. Break out of a case if he pages. He will mail questions to our houses rather than have the letter put in our hospital mailboxes, just to see if we are keeping up with our mail at home. It didn't sound like the Dr. Organ that had calmed a roomful of nervous interns. And, looking around, everyone appeared seasick.

Then, Dr. Bradford suddenly boosted our confidence by telling us that we were not expected to know anything. That sounded like a get-out-of-jail-free card to me. All I had to do was say that I didn't know and I would find out the answer as soon as possible. It seemed like the easiest way to avoid trouble when questioned.

As the morning went on, we were swamped with packets of papers describing how to dictate, how to page, how to log cases, how to get pathology reports, how to code cases, and so on.

There were six "take home messages" that day:

1. Dr. Organ never forgets, so don't ever disappoint him.

2. There are stupid questions. An intern should ask a question only if the answer cannot be easily found elsewhere or if it will change the plan of care for a patient.

3. Never lie. An intern without credibility is not dependable, and, therefore, worthless.

4. An intern is not expected to know anything.

5. An intern is expected to learn everything.

6. The clock does not stop.

Number 6 became my mantra. If I make it through this year, the rest of my life will be easy. It had better be.

Bradford read us the description of the perfect intern off his Palm Pilot. The perfect intern knows everything about his patients, shows up early to clinic, is the last to leave the hospital, is always eager and enthusiastic, brushes his teeth before rounds, never needs the bathroom, is never hungry, thirsty, nor tired, is always clean, and answers questions with "Yes, sir" or "No, sir."

Then we went to lunch at a mediocre Mexican restaurant with lousy service. And I didn't brush my teeth afterward.

*

Internship is the first year of residency. The surgical internship is the basis for the urban legends about doctors working 48 hours straight without sleep and then doing a ten-hour case on your mother. These next twelve months were my twelve labors of Hercules. We changed surgical teams and hospitals on a monthly basis, making each month truly its own labor.

But why did I do this? What I was doing here anyway, a million miles from home? I left behind the best girlfriend I'd ever had, my best friends, and my family. That wasn't me; I'm a homebody. I went to college and medical school less than two hours from home. I didn't even think of applying elsewhere.

I am a wimp. An introvert, bordering on agoraphobic, ever since day one. My grandpa admonished my mom for raising a sissy. My mom feared sending me to kindergarten because she didn't think I would make it through the day with a roomful of strangers. Large social situations still scare me. Throughout college and medical school, people thought I was stuck up because I preferred to stay home on a Friday night than go to a bar. They are terrible, awkward places, bars, nothing at all like my living room.

I had it good. I had Rachel and a couple of close friends who accepted my idiosyncrasies, eccentricities, and psychoses. A small group that could play euchre or Pictionary on a Saturday night, Taboo if I could find a fifth and sixth. Friends who encouraged me to keep painting, which meant staying home, probably because they had seen me dance, or, God forbid, heard me sing. My friends would wait to go out to the bars until 11 p.m., well after I went to bed.

In a moment of weakness, some rarely seen, adventurous split personality seized the reins and flung me to Oakland just to see what would happen. It must have been the weather. I left Wisconsin in November to interview there. Maybe I had a seizure. Or maybe I am part of a reality TV show. Sure, there is something fun about the stress of a challenge. But I feel like I'm the goldfish that jumped out of the bowl. Great, I did it, but now I'm screwed. Sissy was right. I'm the kind of guy who still needs eight hours of sleep a night. If the rumors were true, I'd be lucky to get eight hours of sleep a week.

So, why did I do this to myself?

Maybe because I wasn't dating Rachel at the time I made the choice.

Maybe to get away from my Dad.

Maybe because every now and then I have to try something new whether I like it or not.

Okay, those things might explain why I'm on the West Coast; they don't explain why I took a surgical internship. So, why?

14

Answer: I really want to cut people.

In a legal, organized fashion, which is mutually beneficial to the cutter and the cuttee.

Seriously. I'd die of boredom if I couldn't work with my hands. I'd rather be a carpenter than a psychiatrist.

*

The second day of orientation did nothing to undo Dr. Bradford's damage. It killed me to spend my last day of freedom sitting in a high-school desk with my knees hitting the undersurface, sticking to old gum, while listening to an x-ray tech telling me how to order a film. It can't be that hard. And some woman from Employee Health said she hoped none of us smoked because it was bad for us. Oh really?

A middle-aged female physician closed the morning session with a bit of advice. She said, "You are going to be very busy this year, but one thing is important: Remember yourself. Every day, take time for yourself, to keep sane, even if it is just a minute."

I laughed. One minute? Nobody else found it funny. Were they all serious, scared, bored, or am I just easily amused? What sort of fun could you have in one minute a day? Leave that one rhetorical.

I scanned the room—and realized why nobody laughed. My Palm-Pilot-equipped cohorts were too busy playing Asteroids or chess. Losers. I wished I had a Palm Pilot. How many of them went out last night and bought one while I watched Star Wars for the two-hundredth time? What a bunch of dorks.

They got to save the universe from space rocks while I listened to a woman from the safety department tell us, "If you fall and break your leg, report it to the safety office. It is important for later compensation. If you have a traumatic injury and blood is gushing everywhere, go to the emergency room, but report it to the safety office as soon as possible." Did this imply we were to go to the safety office first if our leg was broken as long as it wasn't gushing blood?

No, Dr. Bradford would say, if your leg isn't gushing blood then get the work done. Good interns don't waste time going to the ER unless it's to see a consult.

I wanted to skip out on the day, but I couldn't because after the stupid talks we were going to get our white coats. Getting the white coat meant more than getting the diploma. The guy with the diploma knows how to take medical school tests. The guy in the white coat, well, he's a

15

doctor. He knows how to take care of patients.

A day earlier, Dr. Bradford told us, "when you graduate from medical school, only two people think you are a doctor: you and your mom." A new intern doesn't really know how to take care of patients; that's what residency is for. And they knew this, which explained why an old lady led us to the deepest bowels of the hospital to give us loaner white coats from a dank room full of white coats on racks and in stacks.

And why not? Why rush into giving us white coats with our names embroidered on them if we won't all be here in a month?

PART 1: THE COUNTY HOSPITAL
Chapter 2

The first day. Only 364 left.

And what a great day it was going to be! A beautiful clear sky lit the world. 6:45 a.m. Sunday morning and I was driving to the hospital. You couldn't ask for a better day to spend inside working.

If I have to arrive at an anxiety-provoking destination at 6:45 a.m., I wake up at 5:45 a.m. And during that hour not only do I eat breakfast, shower, shave, dress, and waste a minute or two plucking errant hairs on my face that have escaped the normal shaving zone, but I also have four loose bowel movements. I excelled in running the hurdles in high school solely because I trained at a couple pounds more than my race-time weight.

The two days of orientation didn't prepare me at all. I didn't even know where the Transitional Care Unit was, but I had to meet my team there. More importantly, I didn't know where the cafeteria was. As I scrambled up to the fifth floor, I took time to notice the truly blissful atmosphere of County Hospital. The somber pale walls, best described as institutional yellow, undoubtedly put upset family members at ease. The hallways were just wide enough to convince others to store things (gurneys, carts, cabinets) in them, making two passing people a crowd.

Guess who stood waiting for me in the TCU? Dr. Palm Pilot. The Green Team Chief. There were so many surgical patients that they were divided into two teams, each with different attendings. Our team consisted of Dr. Palm Pilot and three interns. Usually a team had a junior resident, but the program lacked juniors due to "attrition." The chief organizes call, manages the whole team, teaches, organizes and presents at conferences, and performs the major operations along with an attending surgeon. A junior resident—usually a second, third, or fourth year—helps manage the floor, performs operations the chief doesn't want to or doesn't have time for, sees consults, and helps the interns. (See Appendix B for a hierarchy of hospital staff). Without the junior, Dr. Palm Pilot had a difficult job.

Dr. Palm Pilot's real name was Corey. I gave him points for insisting we call him Corey. Someone a few years my senior isn't worthy of being addressed by a title, unless he wanted to be called Dr. Palm Pilot. I would have gladly called him that. He still stood a chance of having Short Man's Complex, but at least he didn't insist we call him

"Doctor."

Evan out-balded Corey, but you could tell he shaved his head. Bald black men don't get that glare the white men get. (Corey could guide planes in with that beacon.) Evan's good looks stood out, mainly because most doctors aren't good-looking. It's all part of becoming a doctor. Subconsciously, our nation tells the ugly kids to hit the books.

Drat, I guess that means me.

One of the few women interns rounded out our service. She had short blonde hair, scant make-up, and big biceps. She looked like a rock climber. One might even think she was a lesbian, that is, if one was into pigeonholing people by looks. Before I could even learn her name, much less her sexual orientation, Dr. Organ reassigned her to another team.

Evan had a smile for everyone. I think he thought we were going to golf the front nine and go out to brunch. "You ready?" He asked it the same way your experienced downhill skier friend asks the first time he gets you to the top of the slope.

I didn't get to answer. We started by "rounding," just as we would start every day for the next year. Rounding means seeing every patient on our service, examining them, checking labs and films, and documenting everything (a.k.a. writing a note) in their chart. After we round we operate, and after we operate we round. The merry-go-round won't stop until the clock does.

The patients in County all had double rooms. A thin curtain cut the room in half, separating Bed A from Bed B. After a thorough analysis, I concluded there was no pattern to which bed is labeled A or B. The beds themselves were slightly more predictable: There was a high likelihood that whatever function you needed, head up or foot up, didn't work.

The walls were the same pasty color as the anemic patients. Corey said the walls were painted that color so you could ask patients if that's what their stool looked like. If they said yes then you would know their gallbladder wasn't functioning. A healthy gallbladder makes your poop dark.

Apparently the hideous decor revolted some nurses to the point that they didn't even go in the room to check on the patients. Corey said that one morning an intern found his patient dead in bed with rigor mortis already set in. The nurse's notes had normal vital signs recorded less than an hour earlier. When questioned, the nurse admitted she hadn't actually checked the patient in hours because the janitors were waxing the floors and she didn't want to walk through their work. The story might have been BS, but the lesson was not, and it sunk in. Always check the patients and don't believe the chart, especially on floor waxing day.

Our service ran a special on drug abusers. Almost every patient had a history of recent cocaine or heroin abuse. One patient suffered necrotizing fasciitis (nec fasc—pronounced "neck fash") from injecting drugs into his buttock. This is the skin infection from the flesh-eating bacterium popularized in the media. Treatment requires surgical debridement, which means you cut off anything that looks dead until you get to bleeding tissue, and then you pump the living tissue full of intravenous antibiotics. This man had had the skin and fat removed from his right knee up to his right nipple, from the belly button around to the flank. Covering naked muscle were sterile, wet gauze pads that had to be changed three times a day. The intern does the morning change. Luckily, Evan drew that straw.

Corey ho-hummed through every patient visit. He had seen it all before, including the hospitalized prostitutes still trying to turn tricks, skulking down the hall pulling their IV pole alongside them, slipping into another patient's room and closing the door. Yes, Corey proved to be a fount of colorful stories. I wondered how much was truth and how much was embellishment, despite his assertions of veracity.

Corey had more than stories; he provided good advice. "Treat every patient that had a major operation as a trauma patient; they have just been attacked by a man with a knife." I envisioned some maniacal surgeon taking broad slashes at a patient with the flair of an artist. That would explain why Evan's patient with "nec fasc" looked like a shark attack victim.

He also reminded us about stupid questions. "There are stupid questions, and you will feel stupid for asking them, but once you know the answer you won't be stupid anymore." I wanted to ask if that statement was supposed to motivate us to ask questions.

When we finished rounding, the other interns got to go home. I stayed, stuck on call. Whoever made the call schedule had it out for me, making me spend my first night of internship in the hospital. I decided to check out my sleeping quarters in the tower prison. I'd be spending every third night there.

A museum back home called Old World Wisconsin was a favorite destination of grade-school field trips. The museum displayed how country folk used to live. An old-time farm had some hands-on chores. Try to churn the butter. Look, homemade candy. The homes had log walls packed with mud.

I had graduated to Old World County Hospital. The hospital consisted of two attached buildings. The old building was 80 years old. The new one was forty years young. Our rooms, outdated patient's rooms, were positioned right above the ER. This made it easy to go to the ER, but incredibly inconvenient to go anywhere else. Being on the fifth floor with no elevator guaranteed me exercise; the Operating Room was on the ground floor of the new building.

Things stayed quiet for a few hours. I found the cafeteria. I read a chapter from a soporific surgery text and took a nap at the end of each paragraph. At 8:00 p.m. I decided to wander down to the OR to get extra scrubs. Then, I figured I would call Rachel and tell her internship was a cakewalk.

If I had known her when I was interviewing, I might have chosen a program closer to home, but I had met her only four months earlier.

I knew the distance would strain our relationship. If I had any doubts about her, I would have just called it off. But, she liked me despite my faults. That alone made her worth keeping. She even tried to overcome them, and I loved being challenged. Occasionally she even got me out of the house. She thought about the world around her and could maintain intelligent conversations. In my experience, it was difficult to find people who could do that. And, last but not least, she laughed at my jokes. I'd pay money for that.

When I lumbered into the OR, the anesthetist asked if I was going to scrub on the upcoming case. What case? I hadn't been paged. I looked at the dry-erase board, where an appendectomy topped the schedule.

Why was I out of the loop? Shouldn't I have seen the patient? Shouldn't Corey have paged me? He had my pager number on his Palm Pilot. Normally a chief assigns the scut work to the intern. Scut is the nickname for the meaningless chores handed to interns that could be done by well-trained dogs. Corey should have called me to have me transport the patient downstairs, or carry the films, or lick his shoes. I shambled back upstairs, feeling worthless.

But when I walked into the ER, Corey changed all of that.

"Do you want to do an appy?"

So much for calling Rachel. "Of course." I grinned my signature boyish grin; the one I'm told gives away my devious thoughts and poker hands. My first day on the job and I was going to get to operate! It didn't seem important that I had never done an appendectomy before. How hard could it be? You just take out the appendix. Here, give me a knife.

"All right, you'll do it and I'll walk you through it," he told me. "Help get the patient downstairs and I'll see you there." He handed me the chart and left.

I bounced down the ER hallway like Tigger. An appendectomy!

My victim, a young black man, had a stranglehold on his pillow as if the pillow had tried to escape moments earlier. "Mr. Chambers? Hi. I'm Dr. Iaquinta." That sounded strange. Doctor. I wished I could just be Sal, but Dr. Organ had advised us to keep it professional. He kept it old school.

Mr. Chambers didn't care who I was; he just writhed in pain.

As I exited the ER, I walked face-first into the door. The door only opened if you put your hand on the bar. It somehow senses skin, so when I pushed it with my hip, it didn't budge, which made it the highest-tech piece of equipment in the hospital.

Seeing your surgeon smack into a door doesn't exactly inspire confidence. Patients tend to discriminate against blind surgeons. Fortunately, Mr. Chambers didn't see my oafishness as a nurse wheeled him into the elevator. I ran downstairs and caught up with him outside the OR.

Corey pulled me off into a side room. "Have you ever done this before?" He whispered it like we were in cahoots to rob a bank.

"Nope," I admitted. "And I have only seen the operation performed laparoscopically, never open. Why are we doing it open?"

"Because there is a lot of inflammation on the CT scan," he replied. "This guy is HIV positive so you are going to do everything very slowly and carefully. DO NOT cut your chief."

"Okay." The butterflies in my stomach woke up. The odds of getting HIV from an accidental stick were less than one percent. But bumbling interns probably had their own set of statistics.

After we wheeled Mr. Chambers into to the OR, we met at the oversized metal sinks in the hallway to scrub. A surgical scrub is five minutes of washing your hands and forearms. Unless you went swimming in a tar pit, five minutes feels like forever. But, the scrub also functions as surgeon chat time. (I imagine a similar thing goes on in women's restrooms.)

Corey turned to me. "What is the most important thing when doing this case?"

I paused, searching my brain for the answer. "That we get out the entire appendix." It sounded important. If part of the infected appendix is left in, the patient could die from peritonitis (infection within the abdomen).

"No, the most important thing is that we do not get HIV. The patient can die, just as long as we don't get infected with HIV."

The patient can die. Harsh. Yet sensible. When rescuing a drowning person, the rescuer must ensure his own safety first; otherwise, there will be two people to rescue. The last thing I want is HIV. No cure. The new drugs were good, but how good? If I was infected, I would have to become abstinent, and I would never have kids. I would probably die of complications within twenty years. (Mom, if you're reading this, don't get the idea that I will have sex before I'm married.)

I followed Corey into the OR with water dripping off my hands. The scrub tech, already sterilely gowned, handed me a sterile towel. I carefully dried my hands, ensuring the towel didn't brush against my non-sterile shirt. The tech held up my gown and I stepped into it. A nurse tied the back of my gown together. Then, the tech held my gloves stretched open and I plunged my hands into them. I was now sterilely gowned.

I probably had six inches on Corey. He asked the nurse to get him a small platform to stand on. I gave him thanks for caring about my back, but that wasn't his interest per se. A surgeon has to be comfortably positioned to do a surgery well, he informed me.

Corey looked at me from across the patient's iodined abdomen. "You can do as much as you want. Just let me know when you are out of your level of expertise." He drew a line with a sterile purple marker on the abdomen halfway between the belly button and the top of the hipbone. The incision site.

"10 blade," he called.

I put out my hand. What level of expertise? A scrub nurse handed "Doctor Iaquinta" a scalpel to start a case for the first time. After so many years of school, it was my first chance to do what I trained (was training) for. Yes!

When that knife touched my hand, my mind stopped. No excitement. No nervousness. Contrary to everything I knew about myself, I wasn't nervous. The knife transformed me into a machine. And a good machine does what it is supposed to, without doubt or enthusiasm.

I placed my left hand on the skin to provide tension for my incision.

"Wait," Corey ordered.

I obeyed.

He showed me how to place my hand in order to provide better traction. "And make the cut in one smooth motion. Go all the way through the dermis."

I incised slowly, out of inexperience and fear of HIV. The knife slid through the skin effortlessly. I didn't get through the tough, white dermis. Making a second pass sounded a lot safer than sinking the knife too deep. The second pass broke into the yellow fat. I handed the knife back and we spread the skin with forceps. I continued to divide the underlying fat with electrocautery. The Bovie electrocautery looks like a pen on a wire, but it works like an arc welder. When I pressed the button, the tip's connection to tissue completed the electrical circuit, instantly charring the flesh. The smell of burning flesh reminded me of my grade-school friend frying ants with a magnifying glass.

In the past, I'd worked with clay, wood, wax, silver, and cloth. The human body didn't compare to any of them. It's a composite of mushy fat, stretchy bands of muscle, and delicate blood vessels. If I didn't immediately cauterize a damaged blood vessel, the operative site would fill up with blood.

Corey led me through the abdominal muscles. "Do what I do." He stuck a clamp into the muscle, and then opened it. Its spreading tines produced a gap in the muscle.

I put my clamp into the aperture and spread perpendicular to his. He repeated the motion. We bluntly dissected a hole through the muscle down to the shiny peritoneum. "When you cut the peritoneum, you have to make sure you don't cut the underlying bowel. Sometimes it's adherent."

Good advice. He pinched a tiny bit of peritoneum with his forceps and lifted. I could see the bowel below it. I mimicked his maneuver and divided the tented peritoneum with scissors.

Pus gushed out of the slit. I suctioned it up. I found remnants of the ruptured appendix tethered behind the right ascending colon. I definitely passed my level of expertise.

"I think I better do this one. It's an inflamed mess. You don't want to get into the bowel," Corey said. It was his polite way of saying that he didn't want to watch me get into the bowel. He removed the inflammatory adhesions, then the appendix. I anticipated closing the wound; I'd had plenty of sewing time in medical school. But then the phone rang.

The circulating nurse pressed the speakerphone button. A man's voice barked, "Corey, when you're done there, come up to the ER to give us a hand. We've got three GSWs."

Before Corey could answer, the phone clicked silent. Three gunshot wounds!

Corey closed the incision with sutures and staples in record time.

Chaos erupted in the ER. An antiquated type of chaos. The scene made me feel like I worked in the third world. Gurneys congested the long hallway that comprised the ER. If all the rooms are full and there are patients lining the hallways, how many of these people require a surgical consultation? As I ran in, a disheveled man near the door said to me, "You would be grumpy, too, if you were in the pain I'm in." I hustled down to the trauma bay.

In a matter of minutes I saw more gunshot wounds than I had in the previous 25 years of my life. Gunshot wounds aren't the big gaping holes you see in Bugs Bunny cartoons. They're just little gouges, as if a piranha took a nibble of flesh. But these nibbles hurt; the men screamed in pain. Nurses and doctors swarmed around them, poking, prodding, injecting, bandaging. I noticed one of the nurses wore combat boots. How appropriate.

A doctor I didn't know delegated to me the job of cleaning and dressing the wound of the black man shot in the armpit. After a hefty dose of morphine, the victim told me the story. The two groups of men had a shootout in their cars while racing through the city. As they battled alongside one another, one passenger, attempting to shoot the car to his left, shot his own driver in the head. After they tired of shooting each other, they swung by the hospital to dump their wounded in the parking lot before speeding off. The man shot in the head devoted the rest of his life to charity: He instantly became an organ donor. And the man shot in the stomach went immediately to the OR for an abdominal exploration.

Corey ditched me to help the trauma chief down in the OR. Anyone with a gunshot wound to the abdomen that penetrates the peritoneum goes immediately to the OR for exploration. If the shot is anywhere else in the body, you stop to look for evidence of a vascular injury that requires repair. Doctors aren't interested in plucking out bullets like in the movies. If it doesn't gush, there's no rush. That's why I hid the armpit bullet wound with a bandage.

I noticed the clock tick past midnight. My second day of internship just started.

Corey paged me. "There's a woman up there who needs a large abdominal abscess drained. Get her ready so we can follow down here." That meant consent her and fill out the volumes of paperwork. Scut.

According to the bulletin board in the ER hallway, she was in the eye room. There must not have been room anywhere else. I entered the eye room only to find a man with a right eye patch dozing in the chair. I backed out into the hallway. I caught a passing nurse who would have liked nothing better than to not talk to me. "The board says she's in the eye room, but there is a guy in there. Do you know where I can find the woman with the abdominal abscess?"

"Try in the back of the eye room." She never broke her stride.

I thought the back door went to a closet.

I reentered the room and swung open the door to find that we were both right. The "room" had enough space between the shelves of supplies to slide a gurney in and still have a tiny aisle alongside it. A woman filled the gurney.

"Hi, I'm Dr. Iaquinta. I'm from the surgery service."

"Mmm." She didn't even avert her gaze from the medical supplies on the shelf a foot in front of her.

She smelled like old sweat. Maybe we could hose her off too.

"I'm here to get you ready for surgery." My name is Luke Skywalker and I'm here to rescue you.

25

"Oh." She was supposed to ask me if I was a little short for a stormtrooper, but to this portly Princess Leia, I was just another doctor.

The chart revealed that plenty of other residents got to drain abscesses from her too; probably the reason for her nonchalant attitude. She saw the paperwork just as I did: as a waste of her time. This lady didn't want the pen, she needed the mighty sword...right across her abdomen. I skipped re-interviewing her and moved on to the focused exam.

A large red spot, about eight inches in diameter, adorned her belly. I felt the pus fluctuate under the tender, warm skin. Swollen, firm tissue surrounded the pus pocket like the crust around a chicken potpie holding it in. I poked hard enough to make her groan.

My freezing fingers woke her up enough to sign the consent form. That's what I hate about doctors. If something hurts, the first thing they want to do is prod it. And to make it worse, my hands are always cold. During medical school I put a pregnant woman into labor when I measured her fundus (the size of her uterus—or belly).

I spotted Corey in the hallway. "I've got that woman ready to go."

"She's going to wait. We've got a guy with ischemic bowel down the hall." Corey strutted past me and I scampered behind him like a puppy.

Ischemic means not getting enough blood flow. If bowel becomes necrotic, dead and rotting, it will become ground zero for a deadly bacterial infection.

We entered his room; it had the quietude and warmth of a morgue. A pale elderly man laid in a gurney so still that I thought we were too late. Where was the attentive nurse or the caring family member? He couldn't argue that he wasn't dead yet; notes from the local resting home said he was non-communicative.

We backed out into the hallway. Corey glared at me. "If you're going to bring me luck this bad all month, I'm not going to make it."

"Sorry," I muttered. Great, Corey dubbed me a black cloud my first day on call. The field of medicine only had two types of clouds: white and black. Black clouds are busy on call; white clouds get to sleep.

The circles under my eyes competed with Corey's. I think mine won. Wasn't he used to staying up all night? The adrenaline rush of virgin excitement had waned and another major case sounded more like a chore than another thrilling episode of "Adventure into the

Abdomen."

Half an hour later, we gowned again. Corey didn't even offer me the knife. In one swift motion he made a large incision down the center of the abdomen from the sternum down around the umbilicus. The speed at which he divided the fat and got into the peritoneum advertised what four years of training could do. He dug around with his hands like a kid rummaging through a toy box. He pulled out a large segment of dusky purple sigmoid colon.

"We have to take everything that looks bad. If anything left behind dies, he's no better off than not having the operation."

I liked his liberal use of the word "we." I imagined I actually contributed to the case instead of just retracting open the wound and holding the rest of the guts out of Corey's way. Anyone could remove bowel. The gastrointestinal (GI) stapler shoots two parallel rows of staples and then a sliding knife divides the bowel between the rows. The stapled rows prevent spillage of bowel contents. Corey passed the stapled segment to the scrub nurse.

Corey lifted out twelve inches of dead bowel and handed it gently to the scrub nurse, who set it into what looked like a plastic yogurt container. I would have preferred it if he had thrown it to the ground with disgust. Or better, spiked it and followed with an end zone dance.

We sewed the two loose ends together, reestablishing the conduit. Vóila. Then I watched Corey close the abdomen. I didn't want to slow us down and waste any chance for sleep. We didn't finish until 6:30 a.m. and we still had the abscess lady waiting. We kept her waiting and met up with Evan instead.

Evan looked just as chipper as yesterday morning. He had already seen the other patients. He led us through "speed rounds," which meant looking in at each patient from the door while he updated us on their progress. Then we flew by the cafeteria, where Corey and I stuffed our pockets with anything that could be devoured on the run and hidden if necessary. Once, the idea of eating with the very hands that had been retracting bowels only an hour earlier would have disgusted me. Now I had reached a point of fatigue and starvation where it no longer fazed me. You could have served me a pancake on that piece of dead bowel and I would have asked you to pass the syrup.

At 8:00 a.m. we did the incision and drainage (I&D) on the abscess lady. I had to hold back some of the woman's 380 pounds so Corey could get at the lower abdomen. Why did I have to be the fat holder? Corey amused me with his story of his first day on OB-GYN service as a third-year medical student. He was the fat-holder for a 400-pound pregnant woman ready to deliver. When he pushed back her pannus (a giant roll of fat), a snack-pack bag of Doritos fell to the floor.

I accused him of lying. Everyone's heard that urban legend. He was supposed to guide me; I told him that a teacher should never take advantage of his student's naiveté.

"I swear it's the truth. Now pull tight."

I stretched the woman's belly as taut as I could. Corey slashed across the soft, pink spot on her abdomen. Stinky, thick, yellow pus oozed from the gash. He wiped it away with a towel and then pressed on her belly, milking more out.

"Oh, yeah," he exclaimed while forcing more out.

I felt his satisfaction. He just popped world's largest zit. He released the bad humours like the surgeons of old. There is a surgery adage, "Where there is pus, let there be steel." I wonder what they said before there was steel.

The stench hit our noses. I mentally persuaded myself not to gag. The anesthesiologist pulled a bottle of mint oil out of her cabinet. She wetted her fingertip and touched all of our masks. The strong smell of mint mixed with the foul stench of pus ensured I'd never eat anything minty again.

After we finished, we started the day's scheduled cases. For these, one of our attendings would be present. An attending was a hospital staff surgeon, the big boss of the service and, at the same time, one of Dr. Organ's underlings (see Appendix B). They didn't round with us often, but they kept in constant contact with Corey to know how all the patients were doing. We had two attendings. I hadn't met either yet.

Dr. Fagan, the vascular surgeon, approached us outside the operating room. He looked up at me with narrow eyes. I would have guessed him to be in his early forties, but he was well on the way to developing the facial wrinkle pattern of someone who is chronically unhappy.

"Dr. Fagan, this is Sal Iaquinta. He's one of the new interns on service."

"Oh." Dr. Fagan grunted and turned away. He grabbed a scrub sponge out of the dispenser.

28

Oh? That's it? Did I have a reputation that preceded me? Was I just another worthless liability? Was I one of thirteen liabilities that stood a good chance of disappearing, making knowing me a waste of time?

"Hello." I didn't offer anything else. I gave him the silent treatment. When I am tired I get really quiet. Sometimes you can't even hear my footsteps.

Dr. Fagan recognized me for the surgical machine that I was, but in this case that machine was a human retractor. He equipped me with different hooks and retractors and positioned my hands one way or another. I imagined myself as a child's toy. The New Intern Doll. Now with Poseable Arms! He can stand in the same position for hours, without batteries!

I don't remember much about the cases, but I had this great daydream. What if I wasn't really here? What if I was an alien anthropologist just using this body to observe the human race? I was studying the healthcare system, and there were others like me—studying teachers in the school system, mothers at home . . .

If that were true, it wouldn't matter that I stood holding retractors for six hours. In fact, an exuberant anthropologist would consider six hours of close quarters work with the indigent population invaluable. I logged Dr. Fagan's idiosyncrasies. He muttered swear words under his breath and scowled frequently, despite having two-thirds of his face covered by a mask.

In the evening we rounded again. Evan grinned; he said I looked like a truck hit me. I felt like it. At 8 p.m. I dragged myself home to bed.

When I told a friend I was moving to Oakland for my surgical training, she told me that I was going to die, referring to the high murder rate. But she was wrong. I wasn't going to get shot, "they" were going to work me to death.

That's how it started. Haze the new guy. Not one minute of sleep. Go to the ER. Go to the OR. Go to the ER. Go to the OR. My first day on the job: thirty-seven hours.

Only 363 days left.

Chapter 3

I once took a road trip alone to Yellowstone Park. A few days into the trip, I realized that I hadn't talked to anyone for two days with the exception of gas station attendants and hotel desk people. No real conversations, merely transactions. These first few days of residency were exactly the same. Almost all conversation consisted of the necessary exchange of information regarding patient care.

Like an anthropologist trying to learn about the tribe, I gathered little snippets of information about Evan and Corey. Clichés get you nowhere. How are you doing? Fine. I have concluded that 70% of the nation is fine on any given day. The remaining 30% are good. What did you do last night? Not much, I went to bed after I ate dinner.

This must be the depersonalization that Army recruits experience. I prefer to be a quiet person, even secretive, down to a fault. But, I deliberately pried to prove these guys weren't robots. I needed to know that underneath the white coats lived real people, unscathed by residency.

I spent most of my time with Corey, which made him an easy target. He preferred to have me assist him in the OR because I had more operative experience than Evan. At the end of medical school I had worked one-on-one with a rural surgeon who taught me how to assist.

Corey showed me pictures of his wife and baby girl on his Palm Pilot. I knew people passed on eyes, noses, and smiles, but I didn't know they passed on foreheads. Nobody will ever mistake Corey's daughter for the mailman's.

Evan's son looked like a Baby Gap model. His afro stretched to the top of the photo and his grin from side to side.

The days quickly shaped into routine—a process made easier by never taking one off. Now that I was a week into it, I knew the when and where of things so maybe I could start taking time to learn the why and how of surgery.

I knew exactly what I wanted to do at 4 a.m. Sleep. But a nurse in the ICU wanted to teach me a lesson, so she paged.

"Hello, I am calling about patient Harry Gerder. He's crazy. Can I give him some Librium?" a nurse told me matter-of-factly.

I flipped through my list. Mr. Gerder. Bowel surgery yesterday. A yellow team patient—the other surgical team. We covered their patients when on call, and vice versa.

"What's going on?" I love hearing about crazy people and their creative misadventures.

"He's talking about people who aren't there and he's asking questions that don't make any sense. He has a history of alcohol withdrawal; he had delusions when he was in the hospital for a surgery in 1988." 1988? I was in eighth grade.

"Don't we have him on withdrawal prophylaxis?" I asked.

"Yes, but I don't think it's enough."

I threw my coat on, patted down my rapidly thinning hair, and dragged myself to the unit. I welcomed the empty hallways; no dodging between lost patients and family members. The dimmed lights gave the hospital that spooky Halloween 2 ambiance.

I walked with firm steps and long strides. I probably stood six-foot-four with my wooden clogs on. My footsteps echoed down the hall like gunshots. I pretended I was someone important. A high-ranking military officer. Darth Vader. I took a couple respirator-esque breaths and hummed the Imperial March.

The nurse greeted me with the order book and a smirk. I didn't like the smirk.

"Wait a minute; let me see the patient first."

Did she just roll her eyes?

I crept into his room. Despite his scraggly hair and confused look, he didn't appear crazy. Grooming falls to the wayside in hospitals. His eyes looked groggy with sleep, not googly with lunacy. His crisp sheets were tucked in nicely; don't madmen twist them during fits?

"How are you doing?" I asked. Mr. Gerder needed a shave. Crazy people are unshaven. Maybe the nurse was right.

"Just fine, ready to go back to sleep," he politely answered.

Me too.

"Okay, um, could you tell me your name?"

"Harry Gerder." That's one point.

"Do you know where you are?"

He straightened his pillow and looked at me like I needed the psych evaluation. "Yeah, the ICU of the hospital." So far, so good.

"Do you know what day it is?"

"It's Friday morning." That's three for three. Mental status: Alert and Oriented Times Three. He knew who, where, and when.

"I asked you those questions because the nurse said you seemed confused. She said you were asking her about someone who wasn't here."

"Yeah, she woke me up out of a dream to check on me. I started asking her about my dream. I was confused."

"All right, go back to sleep,"

I went out into the hall. "Well, what do you think?" She cocked her head to the side and raised her eyebrows.

"He's fine. He was talking about a dream."

Her shoulders slumped and she rolled her eyes, again.

I turned and lumbered back to bed. I rolled my eyes discreetly.

If I couldn't trust the nurses to make an accurate assessment of a sleepy patient, this was going to be a long year. Corey had warned some of the night-shift nurses liked working when their patients were zonked. Sometimes they wanted doctors to facilitate the patient's drowsiness. I don't believe in this practice. I let the patient ask for sleeping pills. If I was stuck in a hospital, I'd be up all night worried, too.

Wait. I am stuck in a hospital. And I am up all night.

Chapter 4

Not only did the attendings depersonalize the residents by giving us generic white coats without nametags, but the patients were also depersonalized. Referring to people by their affliction (e.g., "the appy in 721") is one of the necessary steps to creating a callous doctor.

Maybe I am cynical. Referring to patients by generic nicknames maintains confidentiality. Because when you overhear, "the GI bleeder farted out a unit of blood," you don't know that the GI bleeder is your kid's eighth-grade alcoholic gym teacher. But if we called him Mr. Andersen then you'd know for sure.

*

On Thursday morning after Grand Rounds (a fancy name for the mandatory lecture attended by all residents and staff, one that nobody finds at all grand), Corey asked me to do an antrectomy with him. Corey almost always gave his orders as questions. They weren't really questions because any attempt to decline was met with frowning eyebrows. The rest of his face could be paralyzed by Botox and he would be able to communicate just by wiggling his eyebrows. Those caterpillars could spell out the letters.

I wanted to do the appendectomy in Room 2 instead of helping him remove a stomach, but I didn't say so. I developed my own subliminal answering system for him to catch on to. "Sure" meant I would rather not, "yes" meant only because you ordered it and I know it needs to be done, and "you bet," meant I would eagerly do it. Sure, I'll go see how our crazy, bed-pooping patient is doing. You bet I'll grab drinks from the cafeteria. I know that I went into medicine to help others—we all did—but that eager devotion started to fade soon after my 24th consecutive hour in the hospital.

"Sure," I answered.

"Good, go get the patient down to the OR. He's in ICU 6." He clearly hadn't caught on. Or he knew it was to his advantage to act like he hadn't. He seemed that smart.

I hadn't met the patient yet, but I knew that he had been admitted to the medicine service for belly pain and they had found a large abdominal mass. That's when they consulted us.

I find it awkward and impolite to meet a patient five minutes before his surgery. It's like showing up at the wrong funeral and everyone expects you to deliver the eulogy. The usual response is a raised eyebrow and non-verbal communication that screams, "Who the hell are you? No one told me kids would be performing the operation. Maybe I don't need this operation that badly after all." And after the patient realizes he is too fatigued to verbalize all that, he says, "Nice to meet you. Will you be assisting the surgeon?" That's the polite way of saying, "I hope you're not the wee child who is going to touch me with instruments I've only seen in horror movies."

I didn't bother meeting him. I didn't want to do that to him. Or, less nobly, I couldn't do that to myself. I grabbed his chart as the nurses wheeled him by. The medicine doctors documented him as this:

CC: 38 Viet. M c 4d Hx of coffee ground emesis.

HPI: 4 mo Hx ↓ app. ?wt loss. +N/V -BRBPR, -D/C

Hx. ex-lap / GSW '85.

I can go on, but you get the point. Here's what it means:

A 38-year-old Vietnamese man had a four-day history of vomiting blood clots. (The CC stands for Chief Complaint and HPI is History of Present Illness.) In addition, he had decreased appetite over the previous four months and maybe some weight loss. He denied (we always use "denies" because it implies he might be lying or just plain unobservant) bright red blood in his stool and diarrhea or constipation. He had a history of having an exploratory laparotomy (when the abdomen is cut open to have a look around and fix things up) after being shot in 1985. The chart went on to tell more about his history, the physical exam, and lab values. The accompanying CT scan showed a large mass at the end of the stomach, presumably cancer.

I followed him into the OR. By that point there were a few new faces, all part of the OR team. He shivered in his tiny blue hospital gown as we had him move from the gurney onto the operating table. Surgeons secretly joke the beds are more comfortable in the morgue.

The morgue might have been warmer, too. The room's kept cold to discourage bacteria from growing. The nurse covered him with a warm blanket and put compression stockings on his legs. These help prevent blood clots from forming in the legs.

The anesthesiologist injected Mr. Ten with a muscle blocker and a thick white liquid nicknamed "milk of amnesia." Seconds later Mr. Ten passed out and then stopped breathing—that's what the drugs do. But before Mr. Ten died (I am not exaggerating), the anesthesiologist tilted back Mr. Ten's head and thrust his jaw open. Then she inserted a long curved instrument in the back of his mouth behind the base of the tongue. She pulled the instrument up and away from the patient, exposing the vocal cords. She inserted the endotracheal tube through the mouth and past the vocal cords in one smooth motion. She connected the other end of the tube to the respirator. She gave Mr. Ten a few breaths from the machine while listening to his lungs to ensure air was inflating both of them. Sometimes, but rarely, the tube has inadvertently been inserted into the esophagus and the procedure needs to be redone.

As soon as the anesthesiologist secured the endotracheal tube, the nurse disrobed him. I shaved the hair on his abdomen with a dry razor and collected the loose hairs with adhesive tape. I cringed at the scratchy, dry vibrations the razor made across his skin.

I went out to scrub, where I met Corey and Dr. Fagan, who squinted at me. I think he recognized me from the other day. My existence verified by a squint. Dr. Fagan squints, therefore, I am!

Dr. Fagan didn't say a word so I spent my five minutes scrubbing my hands and thinking about bigger problems. How much faster would the world have to be spinning so that the centrifugal force would be greater than that of gravity, thus flinging everyone into space?

An intern never finishes washing his hands before the attendings and residents have finished. I waited for Corey and Dr. Fagan to gown up before I entered the room.

After we gowned, we shrouded the patient in blue sterile drapes. We directed the overhead lights onto his smooth golden abdomen, shining with Betadine.

In one swift, deliberate motion, Corey cut the abdomen from the xyphoid process (where the belly meets the breastbone) straight down to and around the belly button. I could tell he derived a secret satisfaction from the process by the enthusiastic way with which he made the incision. The incision became a red stripe. I blotted the blood and he coagulated the bleeders with the Bovie. The burning fat smelled like a summertime barbecue, revealing there's a little bit of cannibal in me.

Corey and Dr. Fagan quickly dissected down to the peritoneum and opened it sharply just above the umbilicus (belly button). Amber liquid gushed out, and I sucked it up with the suction catheter. (We call the fluid "ascites" to make it sound fancy.)

As third man, I sucked up fluids, cut suture, and retracted. The job only sounds glorious. Sometimes I could only see the back of the surgeon's hands or, even worse, their shoulders. Dr. Fagan constantly repositioned me so that I was holding the bowel out of his way. I appreciated the workout. But no matter how hard he tried, he was too short and skinny to block me from seeing the action.

The bowel usually floats free within the peritoneum like a bunch of wet noodles in a plastic bag. The peritoneum is the bag that holds the noodley guts. However, after trauma or previous surgery, the bowel will adhere to the peritoneum. It took about a half-hour to cut loose the adhesions before we found the mass.

A grapefruit of a tumor sat at the base of the stomach. It eroded into the stomach, adhered to the liver, and enveloped the transverse colon.

"This is a dead man," Dr. Fagan said. But Dr. Fagan never just said things. His snivelly voice made every statement a complaint. His short stature, bald head, and beady eyes complemented his know-it-all affect, making him the perfect Disney villain. Maybe I had typecast him from the beginning, but he never proved me wrong.

I struggled to believe we had a person on the table. The sterile curtain hid Mr. Ten's head and the table that held our instruments covered his legs. There wasn't a human in sight, just a big bag of innards. We might as well have been mucking around in a satchel full of organs. He stopped being a recognizable human once Corey opened the first incision. You can't describe people by their innards. He's a nice guy, sure, but have you seen his small intestines?

But Dr. Fagan called him a dead man and made him human again. During a case with that rural surgeon at the end of medical school, we opened the abdomen to reduce a bowel obstruction and found tumors covering everything. As we closed the patient back up, the surgeon said, "That case was an autopsy." This was the same thing.

We poked around a little and verified that the tumor had invaded everything. We found the tumor chewed open a hole in the back of the stomach. No wonder he had bloody vomit. I noticed the little green sac—the gallbladder—stuck to the side of the mass at a funny angle. It appeared intact.

"Close him up," Dr. Fagan said.

When someone has an inoperable tumor, you only take a specimen for the pathologist. There is no survival benefit to "debulking" the tumor.

"What about the perforation in the stomach?" Corey asked.

"There is no point, he's a goner. It won't matter. He won't live a week."

His attitude had changed once he knew the patient had little chance for survival. He spoke much faster. He seemed irritated—disappointed that he didn't have an operation to perform.

"But we could close the stomach to avoid a massive infection." Corey's mask covered two-thirds of his face but couldn't hide the concern in his eyebrows.

"I don't think we should try to sew into that tissue. It won't matter anyway. If he's lucky, he'll die tonight. You guys close, I'll write a note."

I sewed the abdominal wound shut. Right or wrong, getting to close excited me. But the excitement soon waned and I found myself disturbed by the thought of a 38-year-old man dying of cancer. Thirty-eight! I wasn't sure I'd be standing in that OR if I knew I was going to die in thirteen years.

"Admit him to seventh floor," Dr. Fagan ordered. The worst care in the hospital.

"Shouldn't he be in the ICU?" Corey asked.

"Why? What are we going to treat him for?"

That bothered me. We didn't know the patient's wishes. Maybe he wanted everything done despite not having a life expectancy greater than a week. The seventh floor was known for "slow codes." If his heart stopped (coded) the usual emergency actions would occur, but at a slower pace. The slow pace was not intentional; the seventh floor housed the new staff, those inexperienced in emergency situations. Corey said the nice thing about staying on the seventh floor was that it was close to a hospital.

"And no blood," Dr. Fagan added.

I felt sorry for the intern on call that night. Interns covered the floor patients overnight. If he coded, the intern would be responsible for resuscitating him. And he would have to give every effort because there wasn't a documented "Do Not Resuscitate" order in the chart. Only the patient can write that order, not Dr. Fagan.

Dr. Fagan had lectured us about treating the patients like family members even though they were "from a different level of society." Dr.

Fagan, would you send your brother to the seventh floor? He had passed up an opportunity to make a man stable for a few days so the family could say goodbye.

I wanted to object, but fear kept my mouth shut. Forget the hierarchical crap. We're not the army. I know I'm an intern, but I have an opinion. This situation takes nominal medical knowledge. Why not sew the hole in his stomach closed? Give the guy a chance to say goodbye. But I just stood there. It's hard to talk openly to someone who can fire you.

Dr. Fagan slithered out of the room.

"How can he do that? You can't deny blood to someone, can you?"

"C'mon, play God. You can do it." Corey said sarcastically. Apparently, he couldn't argue it either.

We finished closing in silence.

I could work hard all year. But these situations would wear me down. Why weren't we doing anything? Was it just his poor prognosis? I needed to know.

There was no one to talk to. We didn't all meet in the evening, sit in a circle, and discuss the day's stressful events. The closest I could come to any sort of meaningful conversation was telling the on-call resident what happened. Which was meaningless; my patient became just one of twenty-six sick patients she'd be covering for the night.

I decided to call my mom. I enjoyed talking to her. At some point during college, my mom transformed from a mom into a friend. It was probably the fall of my freshman year of college. We went to a Wisconsin Badgers football game and she wore an enormous fur coat that hid her tiny frame. From behind us, we heard someone yell, "Hit the fur!" and marshmallows pelted us from every direction. Then a giant wad of cooked spaghetti hit the ground between us. My mom and I just laughed. A real mom would have been grumpy, but we were friends enjoying the ridiculous situation.

My mom's perspective improved the situation. After I told her the story she said, "Well, now you know not to do something like that when you are in practice." I should almost thank Dr. Fagan for giving me such a good lesson.

Chapter 5

Somehow, everything went all right. Our "dead man" appeared to be a regular, living, human being the next morning. Skin closed nicely. The nasogastric tube sticking out of his nose hardly sucked out any blood overnight. Unbelievably, he denied pain.

His wife spent the day cramped onto the narrow bed next to him, crying. She didn't know enough English that I could communicate with her. Maybe that was better; I didn't know the right thing to say. I could at least look at her with sympathetic eyes.

One of the hospital's translators assisted Corey in discussing what they had found and his poor prognosis. Mr. Ten and his wife agreed to the DNR (Do Not Resuscitate) orders. Afterward, we wrote orders to take out the NG tube and feed him whatever he wanted, a last meal of sorts. Most people can't eat for five days after any sort of bowel surgery, but he amazed us with his appetite. He didn't act like a "goner."

*

The fourteenth day. My first day off. I slept in. I woke and showered by 6 a.m.

By 7 a.m. I felt guilty for not working. Evan and Corey were rounding. I should go help them out for a couple of hours. It had taken only two weeks for me to forget how to do anything except practice medicine. I am well on the way to becoming a great surgeon. I only need to lose the ability to converse with the common man and start a collection of old surgical instruments.

Instead, I decided to do something exciting. No telling when my next day off would be. I went grocery shopping, got a haircut, and had my brake pads replaced on my old Honda. When I returned home I found my pager rattling across my kitchen counter. I called the number just to say I wasn't on call.

"Hello, Doctor?" A woman asked.

"Yes."

"I am calling about your patient, Mr. Ten, in room 7231. He died this morning."

"Okay. Thanks."

I flopped onto my old futon. So that was it. At least his family got to say goodbye. And he had that last meal, pain-free.

How personally was I supposed to take this? Someone just died.

Was it horrible or just part of the job? Should I be sad? Should I dissociate myself from this? Will it wear me out? Is it wrong for it to wear me out, or is it wrong if it doesn't wear me out?

If I take it too hard, I will burn out. But if I lose my compassion, I will be a failure as a physician. Sometimes compassion is the only thing a patient wants and understands.

An alien anthropologist would be disassociated from the event. A human died. That's what Dr. Fagan did. It's the easy way. Humans are prone to taking the easy way. The dark path is easier.

But how will I know the way?

Chapter 6

A swarthy fourth-year resident stopped me in the hallway. I hadn't worked with him, didn't even know him, but whenever I saw him I imagined him plowing me over on the rugby field.

"I see you got your hair cut as short as the rest of your team," he said.

"Yeah, I decided to quit and join the army."

Corey was nearly bald, Evan clean-shaven, and I was now half a centimeter away from them.

"It's the same thing. I have a friend in boot camp, another in prison, and I'm here. I figure we're all living the same life."

I grinned. All three had regimented lives, and in all three situations, the higher-ups did their best to make the people under them unhappy.

Corey proved to be an exception. He enjoyed his work. He took pride in his ability to juggle tasks and efficiently complete them. His naval training augmented his anal nature, creating an extremely organized individual. He managed Evan and me like extensions of his own arms. The two of us gladly worked as parts of a well-oiled machine because Corey never talked down to us, but instead tried to bring us up to his level.

Attendings keep a lookout for camaraderie and promptly destroy it. No longer would the ICU resident or attending help manage our ICU patients because our three patients required too much attention.

Dr. Irving, the ICU attending, delivered this information by speakerphone while Corey and I assisted Dr. Fagan on a bypass surgery. Irving reminded me of Cruella, but all silver hair. Tight lips, like she was used to spitting epitaphs. Skinny frame. Someone you look at and feel uneasy, even if they were offering you candy.

She said, "The only reason I'm calling you in the middle of your case is because your patient in nine is circling the drain and somebody had better come up and take care of him." Click.

I didn't even need to look at Corey' eyebrows to see his fury. It would be impossible for him to finish a four-hour bypass surgery and simultaneously monitor ICU patients. Evan and I didn't have the experience or knowledge to save the dying ICU patient or do the surgery.

"Dr. Fagan," Corey started.

"Go, Corey," Fagan interrupted. "But you better figure out how I'm going to get a chief resident to do these cases with me for the rest of the month."

Corey left to manage the ICU patient. That left me alone with Dr. Fagan to do a vascular repair and reconstruction of a large groin wound. Dr. Fagan whined and moaned. I wanted to ask if he was passing a kidney stone. He said, "I need to operate with someone who knows what they are doing. No offense to you, but this isn't a case for an intern."

Usually when people say "no offense, but…" it means they are going to offend you. I wasn't offended. I already knew that I knew nothing. I had learned that from Socrates.

Unlike Socrates, Dr. Fagan already established that he had no tolerance for teaching. Earlier, in clinic, he had told me to put a patient on penicillin for his wound infection. I started to say what I would write on the prescription, but before I could even finish, he interrupted me and said, "Don't guess and don't ask. Just look it up. I hate it when people ask questions. You don't learn that way. If you want to learn something you have to look it up, read about it. Otherwise you'll remember nothing." That statement excused him from any teaching for the month.

I replied, "Sure."

After he tired of complaining about my ineptitude, he talked about himself. Teaching me about arterial grafts would take away from informing me about his great, new $3,000 mountain bike. He weakly segued into a one-sided discussion about laparoscopic surgery so he could drag me to his office after the case and show me the chapter he wrote on complications of laparoscopic surgery. I also heard detailed information about his stereo system, and how I handled the suture "all wrong." Normally, I love listening to people, but I want to hear about their thoughts, not their possessions.

Dr. Fagan disappeared when the plastic surgeon came in to close the wound with a flap. The plastic surgeon looked like a ruddy farm boy from Iowa, the kid who can't spell "piano" but can carry it across the room. He even acted like a nice Midwesterner. He anticipated a quick procedure, but was duped into doing the case himself with an untrained intern as an assistant. Despite losing half his afternoon, he took the time to give me some one-on-one teaching…without complaining.

Best of all, he stood about a foot taller than Dr. Fagan, so I no longer had to hunch over the OR table.

He let me do the flap, walking me through it step by step. Hannibal Lecter would have been envious. I cut an eight-inch paddle-shaped flap down the side of the thigh and rotated it up toward the groin to cover the patient's exposed arterial graft. This, of course, left a large thigh wound that we covered with a skin graft. I harvested the skin graft with a dermatome. Its oscillating blade shaved off the outer fifteen-thousandths of an inch of skin off the other thigh like a giant razor. This left an 8-by-3-inch "strawberry" that would fill back in with skin over a few weeks. We covered it with gauze. You can rob Peter to pay Paul.

Then he taught me about closing wounds. There are a million different types of sutures all attached to different types of needles. Absorbable suture. Nonabsorbable. Braided. Nylon. Silk. Cutting needles. Taper needles. Different sizes. It turns out the one they call catgut really is made out of intestines, but the cat is short for cattle.

Every attending held a different opinion of every suture. That one breaks too easily. That one spits out of the wound in a month. That one slips. And they all pick a different one as their favorite, even for the same wounds. The plastic surgeon liked to close the skin with nylon (fishing line) because it is strong, non-reactive, and easily removable.

Eight hours later, I had a better understanding of skin grafts, sutures, closing wounds, and what it is like to stand for eight hours needing to pee. (I have a worthless, tiny bladder.)

Meanwhile, Corey stabilized our "drain-circling" patient and met with Dr. Organ to plead for help. We rendezvoused with Evan in the ICU for evening rounds. In the last two weeks we probably hadn't spent more than fifteen minutes a day together. Some "team" we were. They stretched us thin and kept us tired.

"You've got to get married," Corey advised, "otherwise you'll never make it through this."

"Why, so you have someone who can listen to you vent after a day like this?"

"No, so you keep a sense of reality and sanity," he replied. "I go home and look at my daughter and everything seems all right."

"It's nice to have a soft shoulder nearby, too," Evan chimed in.

"Okay. We'll meet at 5:30, see you in the morning." Corey said.

It could have been a serious conversation, but it ran at the same fast pace as the rest of the day. The desire to leave the hospital outweighed any need for philosophical discussion. That's how every night ended.

No wonder it's called a residency. The hospital became my home, my reality. Sure, I called Rachel. I relayed the atrocities I witnessed and she somehow made everything okay. But, cradling the phone between my ear and shoulder didn't substitute for holding her. I still came home to an empty apartment. Six hundred and twenty square feet of pure relaxation.

Rachel was vacationing in Europe, so I didn't have anything to distract me from the insanity that dominated my life. I didn't commiserate with Evan. I thought we would get to know each other, but we only ever met to compare notes, trade chores, and then "divide and conquer."

So I went to bed, alone, with the hamsters running full speed in my head. I couldn't convince myself that a family secured happiness. A month before he died, my dad said to me, "no one's last words are 'I wish I spent more time at the office.'" Too bad he discovered that cliché so late in life. Instead of memories of my dad and me building a treehouse, I got the memory of him apologizing for working 14-hour days for most of my youth. I didn't want to make the same mistake.

So what am I doing becoming a surgeon?

I already told you. I really want to cut people (in a legal, organized fashion etc.).

Besides, the desire to not repeat the mistake my dad made has an alternative solution; I could not procreate.

Working twenty hours a day and having a girlfriend in Europe made that option an effortless reality. But that didn't help me fall asleep peacefully.

Chapter 7

Dr. Organ heard Corey's pleas and we got a new team member, Franklin. Corey informed us that Franklin won Intern of the Year last year—another hard worker would keep the Green Team Machine rolling.

I had met Franklin, not Frank, on call a few days before. He looked like the dopey kid in grade school. His fat cheeks became his neck without any transition. He talked like a washed-up surfer. Cool. Laid back.

So much for first impressions.

He began the day by scolding Evan and me for typing up our census incorrectly. "You guys need to put in the cases for the day. And this isn't how Corey wants it set up." Never mind that Corey set up the census sheet.

"Sal, go discharge the patients on the seventh floor," Franklin barked. "Evan, transfer the guy in TCU 5 upstairs. And make sure there are labs for tomorrow morning." Then he disappeared. In a matter of minutes, he had replaced two weeks of teamwork with a militant hierarchy.

Evan gave me a silent shrug and headed for the TCU.

*

The clinic at County Hospital was a war zone. Clinic started at 1:00 every Tuesday and Thursday and the bodies started piling up at noon. The waiting room became a battlefield as people struggled for position in the first-come-first-served line. Every time I opened the door to call in a patient, there are twice as many "wounded" as before, all with hopeful eyes pleading "call my name." By 5:00, their eyes were shooting bullets that said, "You better call my name next."

Any way I went, I ran into trouble. Here was a Chinese man with widely metastatic cancer. Last week we did a bypass surgery that attached part of the small intestine to the end of his colon. This allowed digested food to circumnavigate the part of the large intestine that his cancer blocked closed. Surgery couldn't cure his cancer, but at least he could eat and excrete. He needed his staples removed, and he still hadn't received a General Medicine appointment for his newly diagnosed hypertension or an Oncology appointment to discuss chemotherapy.

Maybe these appointments weren't important. He had widespread colon cancer. But, as Corey so eloquently stated, "It would be poor form to have him die of a hypertensive stroke before his cancer killed

45

him." And, "We usually give someone the option to go home and die or go to Onc (Oncology) to be poisoned to death."

The nurse helping me couldn't call to make him an appointment. In her words, calling for appointments was "not in her job description." She clarified that she was "a nurse, not a receptionist." Apparently eating Twinkies while working was in her job description. Whoever invented "job descriptions" should be drawn and quartered. Couldn't she just be there to help?

I called the medicine clinic myself. After being put on hold for five minutes, I got to talk to a real person. I could have seen a patient in those five minutes instead of watching Twinkie-nurse suck the cream out of the middle and eat the yellow sponge cake last.

"I need an appointment for a patient with new onset hypertension as soon as possible."

"Our next available appointment isn't until the end of September," the woman replied.

"The patient needs to be seen before then." He won't be alive then. "The medicine team saw him in the hospital and gave permission for an overbook appointment."

"Who's the patient?"

I gave her the name and medical record number.

"He's not in our system," the woman told me in a voice that conveyed that he does not exist and, therefore, does not need to be seen.

"Well, I still need an appointment."

"Who is this?"

"This is Doctor Iaquinta calling from the Green Surgery Clinic."

"Oh, okay. I can put him down for an appointment tomorrow morning, what time is good for him?" she asked. What was going on here? I went from September to tomorrow?

"How about eleven?"

"That's good. Just tell the patient to show up at ten to sign in."

"Thank you very much."

I leaned against the counter, dumbfounded. Either someone had shot her with a mind-altering ray gun, or my doctor status changed her position on the availability of appointments. And I knew there weren't any mind-altering ray guns on this planet. I've looked. I didn't want to

46

be the doctor that threw around his title, but apparently I had to. (Don't worry, you won't hear the maitre d' calling out "Doctor I" at the restaurant.)

Then I called the Onc clinic. The same magic didn't work twice. I only got a "guarantee" he would be called soon.

No time for celebration; millions of people needed our attention. We tried to see as many as possible. Five minutes a person. Less. But some were "time bombs" waiting to go off. The next woman needed more than five minutes to diffuse the situation.

She greeted me with a thick odor. It wasn't quite rancid, but it was yesterday's chicken trimmings.

She completely concealed the chair she sat on. She offered me a pudgy hand as I introduced myself. Ace bandages covered her legs below the knees. The smell emanated from under those bandages. A small puddle of clear, yellow fluid collected on the tile floor below her feet. It wasn't urine. The liquid dripped off the bottom of the bandages. I wish I were anywhere but here.

I asked her if her regular doctor had referred her to us.

"No, I just knew I needed to see a surgeon."

"Who has been treating you until now?"

"I have. I went to the doctor five years ago when I got the first ulcer and he just wrapped my leg in bandages. I figured I could do that myself without coming to see the doctor, so I did." She finished pulling her blue stretch pants above her knees. I waited for the elastic to snap. Both legs had old, overstretched Ace bandages wrapped around them. Fluid saturated the bottoms of the bandages.

"For five years?"

"Yeah." She cocked her head sideways. Duh, anyone can wrap her own legs.

"Do you get short of breath at night?" I suspected she had heart failure. I took a seat on the wheeled stool next to her and pulled the curtain closed.

"No, but I can't get a good night's sleep 'cuz I always have to get up and pee."

I explained to her that the water in her legs was getting back into her system and then being urinated out.

47

I couldn't put off the exam any longer. My secret wish that a tornado would whisk through the clinic and sweep me, or her, away, hadn't been granted.

I gloved up and began unwrapping her legs. Giant ulcers covered her legs from the high shins down to the ankles. They had eroded away the skin and subcutaneous fat, leaving only muscle and granulation tissue, which is the newly formed capillaries and connective tissue that grow in an open wound. Patches of a slimy yellow film covered the pink muscle, like on a chicken. Thin fluid wept from the exposed muscle and collected on the skin ridges of her ankles before dripping to the floor. No wonder it was tile; it needed to be wiped clean with ease.

Her legs were fat at the knees—about 18 inches in circumference—but the lower legs looked like piranha had been chewing on them. The step-off below the knees went in an inch, all the way around. I wanted a camera. I suffer from a twisted fascination with the disgusting. A single photo of her legs would satisfy my requirement for revolting myself for years to come. And, I'd enjoy making my friends vomit.

I couldn't do anything for her venous stasis. The blood that flowed down to her feet couldn't get back up her legs. The pooled blood allowed the water in the veins to leak into the surrounding tissue causing edema, or swelling. Her swollen feet and legs couldn't withstand the stretching, making them susceptible to skin ulcers. Minor trauma damages the skin. And without the nourishment and protection of normal blood flow, infection sets in. Now she had no skin and no subcutaneous tissue, but even worse, the plexus of veins that help return blood to the heart, the ones wealthy women get lasered, were gone. Now she relied only on her deep veins.

I cleaned the tissue and rewrapped it. A skin graft wouldn't take to such unhealthy tissue. What she really needed was to lose a hundred pounds, which would make it easier on her blood vessels. Then maybe a graft would take. But that probably wouldn't happen. After I told her we didn't have a quick fix for her problem, in fact we might not have had a slow fix, she left as dissatisfied as she did five years ago. So, somewhere out there lurks a woman with zombie legs.

After clinic, Corey and I did lightning rounds alone. Franklin was checking on a patient for Corey and Evan had already been dismissed because he only had one patient.

Corey told me not to worry about the zombie-legged woman. We couldn't do anything. He suggested I go home and have some fun; we

48

were done and it was only six p.m.

I tried to believe him but I felt like we were leaving a wounded soldier to go off on her own.

Chapter 8

The next morning Evan and I crossed paths while pre-rounding. "Your boy is all ruffled up; something about you leaving last night without telling him."

"Huh?"

"Franklin stayed here later than you last night. I got an earful about it."

"If I did something wrong he should just tell me." I don't care for grapevines. Besides, that turd-burglar was missing when we rounded.

"Don't worry; you're all good with me. He just wants you to recognize the chain of command." There we were, back in military mode.

Franklin didn't show up for morning rounds. He didn't answer our pages and no one answered at his house. Corey warned, "It will happen to you, too. You'll be scared shitless after you sleep in once because it was so easy. Then, you'll never do it again."

Franklin showed up five minutes before morning conference started, scruffy and panting. "You guys meet me in the cafeteria after conference for a little meeting." No hello. No good morning. Just glaring eyes. He was probably mad at me for not setting his alarm clock.

Evan and I waited in the cafeteria for twenty minutes. Twenty minutes hadn't been wasted in the last two weeks.

I paged Franklin and he answered his page with, "What's up, buddy?"

"Not much; Evan and I are waiting for you." I hate when people call me buddy when they aren't my buddy.

"Where are you?"

Was he kidding? "The cafeteria."

"Oh, I'll be right down there." He hung up.

I watched Evan push the remnants of his runny eggs around his plate for five minutes before Franklin joined us. "I think your boy enjoys having underlings to boss around," he surmised.

"Here he is," I muttered.

Franklin strutted up to the table and flopped onto the chair next to Evan.

"Okay, we've got to have a discussion," he barked. "Things need to change around here. First of all, you don't leave until you talk to me." He pointed a pudgy finger at me.

"I'm sorry, I didn't kn—," I started.

"It doesn't matter, don't do it again," he interrupted. "I had to help Corey with a case last night because nobody was around, and I wasn't on call. There is no reason either of you should leave before I do unless I give you permission."

I saw out of the corner of my eye the two interns at the other end of our table exchange comical glances. They got up and left. Lucky them.

"We are a team. If you finish your work, you should call me and see if there is something you can do."

Wait. Team? Teammates don't talk down to one another. A true team does not have to acknowledge a hierarchy. A true team might have players that are more vital than others, but no member of the team feels the weight of their position. Franklin making us feel piddly wasn't exactly in the spirit of The Team.

"Our primary job is to make Corey look good. This program is fucking malignant. Now you guys lucked out in getting the nicest chief right off the bat. Other people aren't as nice as him."

Yeah, like YOU! Later conversation with Evan confirmed he had the same thought.

"The second thing is that you guys need to birddog the OR. I will tell you the day before what cases you can go to, and when one of you is in a case, the other takes his pager to answer his calls. Then, toward the end of the case, you come in and write the note and the orders."

I couldn't look at him as he yapped his orders. His chubby, ruddy face plumped on top of his thick neck reminded me of Jabba the Hutt. How could I take Jabba the Hutt seriously? He didn't want to work with us; he wanted to work us.

"Forget about each following the patients you admitted on call. You two follow everyone. That way if one of you is in the OR with Corey and one of the attendings wants to round, you know about every patient, because it's going to happen. You don't want to look stupid and say that YOU don't know about a patient because the other is following him. You need to birddog the patients, make sure they got their labs drawn." He droned on with more and more minutiae and used the word "birddog" at least three more times. How I grew to loathe that word.

After he left, Evan and I shared smiles.

"Intern of the Year, my ass," Evan said.

*

I escaped Franklin's wrath to join Corey in the OR, where I performed my first amputation. I lopped off the infected forefoot off of a man with peripheral vascular disease secondary to diabetes.

I used to think that bad luck caused trips to the hospital. When I was six, I fell while rollerskating and broke my arm. That was bad luck. The stitches in my knee? Bad luck. Millions of kids fall everyday while playing; only a few unlucky ones go to the hospital. I applied that logic to the entire nation.

Now that I'd spent a few weeks there, I was an expert. And, in my expert opinion, people did not take good care of themselves. Look at diabetes: It plagues our nation. Uncontrolled disease damages multiple organs. But control requires constant monitoring. Patients must watch their diet and tailor their insulin doses to maintain a normal blood sugar. It accounts for more medical costs than complications of cigarette smoking.

Many people don't succeed in controlling it. A common long-term complication of diabetes is peripheral vascular disease. And just like the zombie-legged woman, the decreased circulation to the feet makes them susceptible to infections. And when they get infected, the antibiotics can't get through the poor circulation to the site of infection.

Diabetes is the most common reason for amputation in the United States. Amputations are an intern-level case, which means a monkey could do it.

I found myself stepping out of a horror movie and into the OR. The nurse put a large blade in my right hand and slapped an oversized forceps in the other. I grabbed a toe with the forceps and cut through the joint with the knife. I tossed it into a metal basin.

Clunk.

I attacked the next toe in line.

Clunk.

Those poor toes. He'd never tiptoe again.

52

Clunk.

He'd never get home late at night and pull off his new socks and pick the sweaty fuzz out from between them.

Among the troubling thoughts of never playing "This Little Piggy" again, I realized how truly powerful a physician could be. I convinced a man I met yesterday to let me cut off part of his foot. What rational man would let someone cut his toes off? What rational man would want to cut someone's toes off? Anywhere else in the world, I would be arrested for this. Anywhere else in society, I would be sent to a psychiatrist if I told someone I think they should let me cut off their toes. But there I stood, hacking away, watching them fall one by one into a steel basin. Clink. Clank. Clunk.

Corey told me to keep cutting. We needed to get to healthy tissue. I looked at the main body of the foot. My gut, my conscience, and my sense of morality all tried to tell me to stop. I had to force my body to do something my brain opposed. The last time I had to overcome the same sick sensation was when I was ten, stuck at the dinner table with the insurmountable task of eating cooked spinach. That didn't go well.

The scrub nurse handed me a rongeurs, a fancy name for oversized wire cutters. The wire cutters deserved a fancy name; they were stainless steel and cost more than my used Accord. I took hold of a chunk of bone and squeezed.

Crunch.

Disgusting. I wish I hadn't thought of gagging on cold, cooked spinach.

But absolutely necessary. Surgery, not spinach.

After the operation, the patient asked me if he would be able to kick a sixty-three-yarder. I admired his ability to keep his sense of humor. Maybe it affected me more than him. Maybe I'm the one who will lose my sense of humor.

I told Corey about our amputee's high spirits. He explained the sixty-three-yarder comment to me. Apparently, an NFL kicker named Tom Dempsey wore a special flat front shoe for kicking field goals. Corey knew everything.

*

Later, Franklin cornered me in the ICU. "It really sucks coming here after a week of endoscopy. My schedule at the VA was 9 a.m. to 2 p.m. Monday through Friday. All I did was scope people. No call and no weekends." He had a far away look in his eyes like he fondly remembered a romantic getaway to Hawaii instead of sticking scopes up people's butts.

"But the Organ-izer destroyed that and now I'm here. They aren't going to give me that rotation back. I just got screwed out of it. So, you can see why I'm not happy. You know how it is, don't you?"

His weak apology for being a butthead didn't win me over. Oh yeah, that sounds rough. Well, if it makes you feel better, go ahead and treat Evan and me like crap. I wasn't about to excuse him; he had already paged me twice since breakfast to meet him so that we could do a "job together" and hadn't shown up. I just did the work myself. Then, he paged me to pass on some jobs that Corey had asked him to do.

Later, Corey paged me. "I figure Franklin's dumping everything I tell him to do down to you and Evan."

"I don't know, probably," I wondered how Corey figured it out so quickly. So smart.

"Well, it's not how I wanted things to get done. But, it is your duty to do whatever your junior asks you to do."

"I know." I didn't expect Corey to do anything drastic or too confrontational. That wasn't his style. And I didn't care; by then, Corey was golden in my book. He knew the difference between right and wrong and he respected people on merit, not position.

"So, did you call GI for that ERCP?" The gastrointestinal doctors performed ERCPs, which is a scope down the throat to look at the pancreatic duct. They can stent small obstructions or remove small stones.

"I tried. She said she doesn't take consults from interns."

"What sort of shit is that?"

"I don't know, she said you had to call her."

"I've never heard of that policy. Give me her pager. Then meet me down here; we can go grab a bite to eat." Click.

Walking to his office was like walking through a minefield. Both paths crossed directly in front of attendings' offices. The best way to go was to cut through the conference room. I sprinted past any open doors to avoid them making a positive ID.

"You ready, man?" Corey's standard greeting. It worked because

54

anytime I saw him, we had to go do something. I wonder if he said that to his wife.

"Sure." We started toward the cafeteria.

"That resident you called, she was an intern until a few weeks ago. I guess she's spent the first few weeks of her second year developing a superiority complex."

I suspected between her and Franklin that such complexes were epidemic.

"But look at that." Corey directed his head toward the pudgy doctor at the end of the hallway.

"What?"

"That's the Chair of the Medicine department in front of us." We approached the stocky doctor at the end of the hallway. He had salt and pepper hair and a matching goatee and wire rim glasses. His white coat stretched over his belly and he had a medical magazine tucked under his arm. The archetypal doctor.

"Dr. Harris."

"Hello, Corey." His greeting contained a question. He knew to suspect something. Surgery and Medicine didn't interact without reason.

"Is it policy for the medicine residents to not accept consults from interns?"

"No."

"Because if it is, it's going to be difficult for me to call in consults while I am operating. My intern wouldn't call a consult without it being discussed with me first anyway."

"Well, it isn't policy. Who's doing this?"

"I don't want to mention any names, but it was the GI service."

"I'll talk to their chief about this." He straightened his medical journals and scurried away.

"Thanks." As we walked away, Corey broke out into a devilish grin. His step had a gleeful bounce as he patted himself on the back for sabotaging the GI resident.

How evil.

Franklin left that night without signing out to the resident on call. That meant that the resident got calls about patients he didn't know about. I imagine it was quite inconvenient because Franklin had two patients in the intensive care unit. He broke his own rule.

If nothing else, he will be interesting to work with and observe for the next few weeks…from an alien anthropologist point of view.

Chapter 9

Franklin tried to burrow under my skin. When he admonished Evan and me, he focused only on me. I think he wanted me to talk back. He knew he could let loose a satisfying berating if I shot my mouth off. But I didn't give him that pleasure. Instead, I learned to look at him blankly with my mouth hanging open as if I was too dumb to know how to breathe through my nose. I ensured I looked like an idiot by avoiding blinking and focusing my eyes a foot behind him.

He reminded me of the senior goalie on the high school soccer team who got his kicks by trying to make me carry his stuff. A smart freshman knows what's good for him. Franklin doesn't know I never gave in. The only way Franklin could break me would be to sit on me. Or even worse, sit on me and drop ants into my ear. I hate the idea of ants crawling in my ear canal.

My odd behavior drove Franklin to interact with Evan more often. Evan wasn't thrilled about the extra attention. He complained, "Your boy is killing me. I'm birddogging the entire hospital."

"Why do you call him 'my boy'? He calls you bro, not me."

"Yeah, what's up with that?" Evan commented on Franklin's choice of slang when talking to our black patients. Apparently, Franklin overstepped his bounds.

"I sure hope getting him has made Corey's life easier," Evan sighed.

*

I believed the sudden schedule change had made Franklin miserable. But being miserable just meant he fit in. The hospital bred unhappy people. Cold people. Nurses that couldn't schedule appointments. Doctors that didn't get personal with patients. Attendings that grunted their hellos.

Franklin fell into their trap. Didn't he read the orientation manual? They wanted to make him a cold, unhappy person.

The manual recommended we address patients as Mr. or Ms. It instructed residents to avoid opportunities for familiarization. "Being of a first-name basis with patients is not necessary and demonstrates a lack of respect."

My medical school spent four years trying to create physicians that would seem like real people. The mentors encouraged us to learn about my patients, their hobbies, and their home lives. Get on a first-name basis with them. Speak to them in their language. Make the patients participate in their health care. Patients are not sick pets treated by white-coated strangers who speak a foreign language.

All of their little rules and sufferings were part of the initiation. Crossing each hurdle meant that you were one step closer to being a really special person. A surgeon. Residency is a good way to alienate yourself from the rest of society and, at the same time, elevate yourself above everyone else. I guess that is the goal of any would-be successful cult. Forget about killing a goat, we get to hold a beating heart in our hands. We are all gods!

Three weeks into it and I knew that I didn't belong.

I documented my feelings by painting a picture—not all in one day.

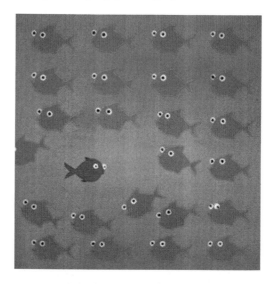

I am not an artist. I started painting on a whim during the last year of medical school. And I started with the easiest of mediums.

Acrylic paints accommodate the busiest of schedules. Acrylic dries in minutes and the brushes clean quickly. This means that you could paint only ten minutes a day and still have a good-looking painting, especially if your paintings look like cartoons. Oils take days to dry and are far more tedious to clean. Acrylic forgives; it is so opaque that you can cover your mistakes, not like watercolors where any overlap sticks out like a sore abscess.

Chapter 10

I returned to the trenches. The clinic looked like a barracks. Curtains divided the large room into cubicles, making privacy impossible.

I found myself talking to one patient, trying not to wince as I listened to a man on the other side of the curtain scream as Evan repacked his wound. I watched my patient fidget; undoubtedly worried he'd be tortured next. I could have made him pass out if I told him I'd be right back with a hot poker.

Sometimes patients forgot that they weren't in a private room. Evan came out of a cubicle into the hallway when we heard his patient call out, "I've got hemorrhoids and warts on my butt, too!"

The closed curtain saved us. Evan could grin silently, but I had to bite my wrist to stop from bursting with laughter. I never was good at stifling laughter. If I held it in too hard it made me fart.

Dr. Francis Ford Coppola was our attending surgeon du jour. He wasn't really Francis Ford Coppola, but he wasn't Dr. Fagan, aka, Dr. Snively either. But his large frame, big glasses, and slicked-back hair reminded me of Francis Ford Coppola. He joked we worked at the Center for Advanced Disease. Corey smiled politely, as if he heard it from him numerous times. Attendings must love their job. Every year brings in fresh meat to grind into hamburger and a captive audience that hasn't heard their jokes.

Anyway, back to Dr. Coppola's point. In middle-class suburbia, people get their gallbladders out as soon as they have belly pain. But here we compiled a waiting list of 12 people who needed to get the gallbladders removed because of gallstones. We just didn't get enough OR time to get things done promptly. Some patients would return to the ER with acute pancreatitis because a stone occluded the common duct, because we didn't do their surgery on time. Then, we got to take care of advanced disease. Pancreatitis can be life threatening, take weeks to resolve, require numerous operations, and cost taxpayers hundreds of thousands of dollars. The people who clamored for nationalized healthcare had better be wary of what they might get. After all, County is government-run healthcare.

In the Old World Hospital clinic, I met a man with a testicle the size of a small cantaloupe. I could hear gurgling bowel sounds when I put my stethoscope on it. He had a hernia large enough for a loop of bowel to get down into his scrotum. Diagnosis: gutzinnutz. I made that one up myself. I wanted to share my joke with Dr. Coppola, but he had already disappeared. Attendings excel at vanishing.

Less than an hour later, a Filipino woman complained that a lump in her belly had appeared after coming back from the Philippines two weeks earlier. She had no other complaints, just an abdominal mass. My mind raced with fantasies of exotic parasites balled up under her skin. I gladly rolled up my sleeves to examine her.

I resisted giving her a good tickle and gently felt her stomach. I found a firm mass extending from her liver down to her pelvis. Once again, it was the size of a cantaloupe. It bounced around in her peritoneum like an ovarian tumor—I had felt one once before, in medical school, which pretty much made me an expert of such things. I silently hypothesized the tumor had been lurking there longer than she thought. Cantaloupe-sized lumps don't appear overnight.

Unfortunately, I wouldn't ever find out the truth. By the time she would return for follow-up after her CT scan, I would no longer be on the Green Team. If I were lucky, she would be presented in conference.

I secretly enjoyed clinic when it ran smoothly. The scenes flowed like the video montage to pop music in the middle of a movie. Everybody looked like they were having a gay ole time changing dressings over skin grafts, listening to gurgling testicles and palpating abdomens. The interesting patients were a fringe benefit. It's not every day you find fascinomas and horrendiomas. Or gutzinnutz.

The day provided me with enough stories to entertain Rachel that evening. She had finally returned to Wisconsin after two weeks in Europe. We exchanged stories on the phone until I passed out from exhaustion.

After we hung up, I wondered if I missed her as much as I should. I had been lugging myself home every night and falling into bed. I never sat around thinking how nice it would be if she were there; I just went to bed. Could working so hard be ruining our relationship? What a horrible thought. It was much easier to find work than love. After all, everybody had a job. I tried to think about it more, but fell asleep instead.

*

When I woke up, I knew I missed Rachel. I didn't have to try to think about it. She just kept popping into my head. And why shouldn't

I have missed her? If I didn't love her, I wouldn't have looked at her picture while talking to her. Rachel embodied "woman" more than anyone else I had ever dated. Not that I dated farm animals before I met her. She not only was more mature, but she looked more mature. She looked like a businesswoman in the movies; tall and svelte. She had a slender nose and fair features, almost like an Englishwoman. And despite being a bookish medical student, she wasn't ugly...an exception to the rule.

I stink at photography, but this one shot made me proud. I caught Rachel grinning at the camera with her straight, blonde hair blowing across her face, laughing because she had just said, "Hurry up and take the picture, dork." Supposedly photos look best when you catch people doing what they love, in this case, harassing me.

When I was in grade school I had complained to my mom that a girl at school routinely made fun of me. She told me, "When a girl teases you, it's probably because she likes you." Well, it wasn't long before I realized that every girl in school liked me. Rachel's insults proved the streak was still alive.

Turns out my mom is sometimes right. I had a girlfriend that knew I was dork, often called me a dork, but loved me anyway. Hopefully, my job and our distance apart wouldn't destroy us.

I wondered if the distance between us might prove to be ironic, if what brought us together might be the very thing that broke us up. If I hadn't been leaving the state, I doubt I would have had the courage to ask her out. I knew that if she said "no," it wouldn't matter, because in a few months I'd be escaping to California with my tail between my legs.

Normally, I would spend a few weeks daydreaming about asking a girl out on a date. My hands would sweat profusely if I actually went near the phone to try to call her. Then, I'd spend a few weeks convincing myself that I'd built her up in my head and she was not worth asking out. Meanwhile, she'd start dating someone else.

I'm quite apprehensive about conscious people. If you were sitting alone on a bench, I couldn't walk across the park to meet you. But if you were lying asleep on a table, I would eagerly cut out your appendix without so much as a handshake.

So, in a moment of bravado I found myself ringing Rachel's doorbell, despite having met her only once and her not having appendicitis. And after a few minutes of awkwardness, which she sensed the moment she opened the door, she agreed to go out on a date, even though she wasn't looking to date anyone because she had just ended a long-term relationship. She later admitted that the only reason she said yes was because she knew I was moving. What could be the harm of hanging out with me?

Sucker.

With the freedom to be relaxed because we knew we were going nowhere, we had a great time. We went hiking and picnicking. We ate barbecued ribs. And then, bam, we fell in love.

Chapter 11

In between working with egos, bowing to bosses, inhaling hospital cafeteria cuisine, and changing bandages, I got to do some cool things. Sure, I didn't cut people as often as I wanted, but they gave me chances here and there.

I performed my first laparoscopic surgery—that's when we operate through small ports in the belly with tiny instruments and a tiny camera. It makes surgery into a video game. I watched my instruments on a television screen while dissecting away tissues with tiny scissors. I activated the electrocautery with a foot pedal. I clipped small blood vessels with miniature staples.

I couldn't believe those fools let me operate. When I went to Old World Wisconsin I didn't get to drive a tractor. Where were the limits? Sure, I went to medical school, but how did that make me qualified to do this? We never practiced sticking long instruments into people's abdominal cavities. One wrong move and I could have poked into the liver or perforated the bowel. That would have ended the fun real quick.

I guessed they let me do it because they had Corey to stand over me. The experience reminded me of being six years old and my dad putting me on his lap in the car to let me "drive." Corey directed and redirected me the entire case. "Retract that with your left hand. The world has no great one-armed lovers."

"What?" I cocked my head sideways.

"Use your left hand," he said. "A surgeon always has both hands working. Your left hand should always be helping your exposure or providing counter-traction."

For a moment I felt sorry for one-armed people. Lousy lovers and no arm. How rough could life get?

I yanked the gallbladder away from the liver. I cauterized the junction of the liver and gallbladder, causing the little green sack to fall away. When I pulled the intact gallbladder from the port near the patient's belly button, Corey said, "All right."

I didn't know if he meant I had done all right, or if he meant all right, we were finally done. I thanked him for his patience. He would have finished twenty minutes earlier if it weren't for me. Corey didn't care; he'd done a million gallbladders. One of the saving graces of General Surgery is that one of their bread-and-butter cases is also a load

63

of fun.

Those moments of operating on the edge of my ability were what made internship worthwhile. I had run my dishwasher five days earlier and it still sat full. The only dirty dish I had in the sink was a bowl and a spoon. Every night when I came home I had a bowl of soup. Every morning I grabbed that same bowl and ate my cereal out of it. For five straight days I had sat at my kitchen table, my posture a perfect letter "C," hunched forward reading a surgical textbook while rapidly spooning food into my mouth. My mom would kill me if she saw that. If I was going to live like this, I had better get to do something fun during the day. Just as the woman had told me during orientation, I needed to get my minute.

The minute was supposed to be for myself, but I'd give it up for the chance to operate. There was something peaceful about the non-scary parts, almost like working on an art project. Corey clearly enjoyed it too. He told me, "You can go shoot hoops anytime. But, Michael Jordan will never be able to operate." I couldn't agree more.

Chapter 12

I went to see the patient with nec fash (necrotizing fasciitis). He healed so slowly that he'd probably be in this residency longer than I would. We had skin-grafted his back the day before, so he had to lie prone for another four days. If he rolled over he would scrape the graft off.

"How are you doing today?" I examined the edges of the bandages. I didn't smell the musky odor of infection. Good.

"I'm doing fine."

See, everybody is doing fine. This guy is lying in bed, unable to roll over, missing a third of his skin, and he was doing fine.

"Can you move my water closer?" he asked. Someone had pushed his tray table away from the bed. I slid the table and cup toward him, but stopped just out of his reach.

He stretched for it but fell short and rolled his eyes up toward me.

I gave him a big smile. Then I pushed the cup into his open hand.

He smiled. "You know when I first met you I thought you were a stiff, but you're a real card." He laughed.

One of my goals as a doctor was to make every patient laugh. But, I had been too busy transforming myself into a healthcare automaton. I didn't want to change my personality to become a surgeon.

Did I have to?

*

I grinned all the way to Dr. Organ's office. I had a private meeting with him. During orientation he had requested that each of us make an appointment with him so he could get to know us. Corey's intro speech scared me into believing Dr. Organ would be keeping tabs on who stopped by.

I waited outside his office, anxiety-free. Usually I would have stopped by the bathroom for such a momentous occasion. But not today. My feeling of insignificance provided me a comfort blanket. A shark like Dr. Organ wouldn't waste time on a minnow like me.

He called me in. Classical music emanated from the corners of his spacious office. I spied the white speakers hiding on the wooden bookshelves among volumes of surgical textbooks. He offered me a seat.

He called his secretary to bring in a copy of my personal information.

I sat quietly. No speaking unless spoken to. Less chance for error that way.

"Are you working too hard?" he asked.

I couldn't believe it. His first question was a trick question. "Yes" meant I was complaining, and "No" meant I wasn't working hard enough.

"I am working hard, I'm busy, but I am surviving."

"Good." He glanced down at my papers.

I passed!

"What do you want to do in five years?" He stopped scanning my file to put me on the spot. He looked directly into my eyes.

I want to be a racecar driver! An astronaut! A fireman? Anything but your resident whipping boy. "I'm not sure. There are many aspects of Otolaryngology (ear, nose, and throat surgery) that I like. That's why I chose that specialty. There are many interesting options." Why am I talking like that? I don't talk like that. Did my heart just pick up the pace?

He returned to the papers. I scanned the office. He didn't have any pictures of his family. I didn't see a single personal item. The room offered no evidence of a life.

"I was in Nebraska at the same time as your medical school's head of surgery. Did you know him?"

"I met him a few times." Is this getting to know me?

"He's a very nice man."

"Yes, he is. Everybody likes him." I hoped I didn't come off sounding like a brownnoser.

"You know, we each work for competing journals."

I didn't have anywhere to go from there. It didn't seem like conversation, just a series of statements.

Dr. Organ talked about his past some more and then said, "It was nice meeting you. You are the first one to come. Every year I tell people to stop by, I am always curious to see who will actually show up."

"Maybe people are intimidated," I offered.

"They shouldn't be."

You didn't hear Corey's introductory speech about you.

We both walked to his door. I started down the hallway.

"You know, this year will be what you make of it," he called after me.

I turned back. "I know. Everything in life is that way."

Chapter 13

That morning we saw a young, black woman with an abdominal cellulitis (subcutaneous fat infection) from shooting black-tar heroin into her abdominal wall. Scars from previous I&Ds (incision and drainages) crosshatched her belly. We were keeping a close eye on her to make sure her cellulitis didn't turn into the nec fasc. Evan's shark attack victim's had.

Corey told her, "Don't shoot into your stomach anymore. *If* you're going to use, shoot into your leg. I can cut off your leg but I can't cut this off if you get a severe infection." He waved his hand across her abdomen. "It could kill you there. And *don't*, whatever you do, shoot into your neck. I can't cut your head off. You can use your forearms, but most people find their arms more important than a leg."

"Okay," she had the wide-eyed look of a six-year-old being admonished for "doing bad."

As we walked out of the room she called after us, "Thanks, Doctors."

Corey pulled Evan and me aside in the hall. "The reason I say it like that is so they understand. Next time they shoot drugs they'll remember this. If you tell them it is a choice between death, an arm, or a leg, they'll choose the leg."

Of course. Because those are the only choices. Where was the ideal world? Where was the social worker that would assist this patient in finding a way to get clean?

These little episodes reinforced the feeling that I worked in Old World County Hospital. Country boy in the big city. Farm boys didn't shoot drugs. They were happy enough with beer.

But that wasn't true either. My little sister grew up in the same small town I did, yet she became a heroin addict during college. It killed me to see these patients. Was Jill showing up in an emergency room somewhere? Did she have an abscess, or worse, necrotizing fasciitis? I feared calling her because I didn't want to hear the drugs in her voice, but if too much time passed without word from her I'd imagine her lying dead in a street somewhere. This sounds melodramatic, but she already had one failed suicide attempt under her belt, so anything was possible at any time.

The uncertainty killed me. I am embarrassed to admit that I had thoughts that it would be easier if Jill had succeeded in her overdose.

Not because I didn't love her, but because if she were dead there wouldn't be any wondering. There would have been no worrying about her relapses or why no one had heard from her in eight weeks. But those thoughts are the easy way out, and I've already established the dark path it easier.

I know...there are places to go for help. But the only way to get an addict to one is if an addict wants to go. Kidnapping remains illegal, even if the cause is altruistic. Which leaves my family with worrying. Worrying about Jill probably took years off my mom's life. No way would Corey's speech make it into the next phone call home.

I kept my mouth shut as Evan and I followed Corey down to clinic. Moments later, the patients upstairs were forgotten and their problems replaced by sixty people with their own concerns.

Corey started the afternoon pleading with the chief clinic nurse and self-appointed father figure of the clinic. We were all his children, whether we agreed to it or not. The fact that he had graying hair and twenty years on us solidified his authority. And his beard and glasses gave him an air of scholarly wisdom, something us young boys of surgery surely couldn't have.

I could hear Corey arguing with him from outside of the curtained cubicle.

The two stood face to face on the other side of the drapes from Corey's patient. The chief nurse retorted in a loud whisper. "Listen, I am a compassionate man, but if a patient doesn't show up for surgery and dies because of it, it is his own damn fault."

What did Corey want to do in clinic? I finished with my patient and peeked into their cubicle. A scraggly man in a flimsy gown rested on the table. I spied a large ulcer on the man's leg. Cancer. I knew immediately he was the patient that didn't show up for his surgery earlier in the week. Corey had told me about his nasty lesion.

Corey argued the way he always argues: adamantly and logically. Neither appealed to our nurse. Corey repeatedly pointed to the large melanoma on the man's leg, insisting that the tumor had to be removed. And our nurse repeatedly responded that it was too large to remove in clinic.

Obviously, Corey hadn't heard Franklin's suggestion of how we should approach our chief nurse. Franklin said he'd "be our man" if we brought him Rice Krispies Treats from the cafeteria.

69

But Franklin was too busy with the Spanish translator, the pretty one he was trying to describe to me the other day. "You know, the one with the nice rack," or was it cantaloupes? Everything in clinic is always the size of a cantaloupe—breasts, tumors, testicles, you name it. Franklin kidnapped her and saw all the Hispanic patients, with complete disregard to the actual order of patients.

I grabbed the chart of my next patient. Anal skin tags. Why do I always get the butt patients?

I explained to an irate middle-aged woman that we only had time for emergency and cancer cases just then.

"I know how this place works; it will take months for me to get these removed."

"You're right, but there is nothing I can do."

She looked at me desperately. "But I had a surgery date that I missed two months ago. Can't I just get another?"

If your hemorrhoids bothered you so much, why did you miss your surgery date? What was so important that you decided to keep your butthole looking like a sea anemone for another couple of months? I was so tempted to say it, but if I did I would be taking a step down the dark side. Rumor had it there were more anesthesiologists back then, but Dr. Organ fired most of them last month for being lazy.

Then she transformed into a monster. Her eyes widened. A long finger with an even longer fingernail pointed at me. She demanded she get her surgery date.

She didn't understand that intimidating me for a surgery date was like begging the janitor at Soldier Field for box seats. I told her to dress while I refilled her prescriptions. It disappointed me that uninsured patients could be so demanding. We were trying to do what we could with limited resources. Telling her that Corey was trying to cut out cancer in the cubicle next door wouldn't make a difference to her and her hemorrhoids. I did the only thing I could. I added her to the ever-growing list of people waiting for surgery and moved on.

My next patient had a breast cyst. By that time, Corey had succeeded in breaking down the chief nurse sans Rice Krispies Treats, and had completed his major operation. So my request for the needles to drain a cyst was like asking for a band-aid.

If you approach a difficult situation knowing you only have a few minutes to accomplish it, it allows you to bypass most of the hurdles.

For instance, being able to hit a small lesion with a needle through an inch of breast tissue isn't something I practiced in medical school...ever. Not once. Oh well, no time to worry about that. The patient waited hours for this moment, so she wasn't going to ask if I had ever done this before. Another hurdle cleared. I focused on properly preparing the site and the needle for the biopsy, which hid the fact that my innards were trying to shake themselves out of any available orifice. Another hurdle narrowly cleared.

I pushed her breast against her ribcage, pinning the mass between my left index finger and thumb. I almost closed my eyes to "use the force." Nothing like the voice of Old Ben Kenobi in your head to calm you down and build confidence. Funny I imagined Alec Guinness cheering me on instead of my dad.

I sank the needle through her skin slowly and smoothly. I swear I felt a tiny pop as it entered the cyst. I pulled back on the plunger. Yellow fluid filled the syringe.

I hit it on the first shot! I performed a victory dance in my head. I had to keep up the appearance that I did this sort of thing all day long, but man did I feel like the kid that got picked to churn the butter back in Old World Wisconsin. Yeah.

The whole thing felt fake. Nothing could be real. How could they let me poke women with needles? How could there be people who skipped their scheduled surgery date, even some with cancer? How could there be drug addicts who lose half the skin on their body? Or had been shooting into their neck because their veins were too damaged everywhere else?

Chapter 14

Every morning at 7 a.m. (except Thursdays), we had morning report. The chiefs of each service presented the previous day's admissions to all of the attendings. Dr. Chi, the trauma chief, started first. Her long black hair and smooth complexion made her look like a high-school student. But when she talked she dispelled that mirage with her cold, business voice.

"Our first activation is a transfer from Community Hospital. He came in with a gun shot wound in the right upper quadrant." This would be under your ribs on the right side of your belly.

"Why was he transferred?" interrupted Dr. Organ.

"Because the patient didn't have insurance."

A resident was using sarcasm during conference? She'd surely be hanged.

"I think you mean because the patient was stable and there were no available surgeons at that hospital," offered one of the two trauma surgery attendings. He looked the artist archetype: curly hair, glasses, skinny. He madly doodled on scrap paper all conference long. I'd have bet anyone five bucks that he'd snap some day.

"No," the trauma resident replied firmly. She wasn't being sarcastic. She was telling the truth.

The doodler explained that it was illegal to transfer, rather than treat, an emergency patient because they didn't have insurance in an emergency situation. He went on to explain that extenuating circumstances, such as not having the necessary surgeon or equipment, would be reasons for transfer. His tone suggested the patient was improperly transferred.

"The patient was transferred at 6 p.m. He was brought to us with a systolic blood pressure of 80." The trauma resident delivered the answer with the calculated speech of a robot.

That said it all. A young man's systolic pressure should be around 100 to 120. Hypotension is a sign of shock. The bullet probably damaged the liver or a decent sized blood vessel and caused internal bleeding. Community Hospital always had a general surgeon in house.

"Why did you accept the transfer, then?" Dr. Organ asked. In a less formal setting anyone else would have asked why she accepted a "dump."

72

"We had no choice. We didn't hear about him until he was in our ER."

"How does a surgical patient get transferred here without anyone speaking to the surgeon?" The trauma attending's face filled with blood. Today just might be the day he loses it.

"The ER physician accepted him."

"They can accept surgical patients without your consent?" If the trauma surgeon opened his eyes any wider we'd have our own surgical dilemma.

"Yes, there is no protocol that involves informing the surgery team." She looked the attendings in the eye when she answered every question, and didn't fidget. I wished I could be that confident.

That got the doodler spinning. He spat out words like "investigation" and "repercussions." Then he turned his focus to scribbling on his scrap paper.

When you get an attending mad, make sure he's getting mad at someone else. Or, have a pencil and paper for him to scribble out his frustrations.

This must have been more of the Old World Health Care display. In the real world, emergency patients wouldn't be transferred just because they didn't carry that hospital's insurance. It's not about money; it's about getting patients healthy, right?

Wrong. If the government's reimbursement for taking care of an uninsured patient made it profitable to do so, why would private hospitals ever transfer a patient?

*

That night we went to a dinner paid for by a drug rep.

Healthcare workers shouldn't receive gifts from drug companies. Pharmaceutical companies spend billions a year on advertising. That's crazy.

In an ideal world, there would be no advertising. Medical products would be used because they were proven to be best for the situation. There could still be reps, but their job would be to supply doctors with the details of their product and the studies that prove its efficacy. It would be more like carpentry. The carpenter doesn't need a rep to tell him to use drywall screws instead of thumbtacks. Advertising isn't necessary for him to choose between a roofing nail and a finishing nail.

He just needs to know what screws and nails exist.

But if advertising didn't work on doctors, they wouldn't take us out to dinner.

I told Corey my dilemma. He told me it was only for our surgery team and the two attendings. They expected me to be there. It was our last hurrah as the Green Team; the month was just about over.

Corey said, "When I was a med student I was the same way. One time I went to a conference where the reps were trying to push the doctors to use Tylenol rather than acetaminophen (generic Tylenol) because the generic counterparts weren't as closely regulated. What sort of bull was that? But there were doctors eating it up. I couldn't believe it.

"But now I realize they provide me a service," he continued. "They tell me about things that I don't have the time to look up myself, or even wouldn't take the time for. Anytime they tell me about the 'new great thing,' I ask to see the papers on it. I check if it was a good, randomized study, and how it compares to the current standard of care. Any good rep has those papers in their briefcase.

"If I can get them to take my wife and I out to a fancy dinner, I go," he said. "I don't have the money to take my wife out to the restaurants they take us to. And if I couldn't bring my wife along, why would I spend my free time going to one of their talks?"

"It still doesn't seem right."

"You will never give anyone anything but what you know to be the best care. Would you ever compromise your treatment plan and prescribe the wrong drug just because it was advertised over a dinner?"

"No." But it might not look that way to other people.

"Right, and neither will I. But, I will take the opportunity to enjoy something nice. I've arranged for us to have a dinner at one of the nicest restaurants around. You shouldn't turn that down."

"Sure," I muttered.

Corey was good at the logical argument, but it didn't change my gut feeling. Maybe Corey was right about the dinner this time, but that didn't mean ugly things weren't going on under the table and I was associating myself with these companies. At the very least, the patients were paying for this dinner.

I set my over-analyzing aside to enjoy dinner. We discovered we were more than healthcare-providing robots. I didn't know that Dr. Fagan liked women with big breasts...so much in common with Franklin. And I got to listen to the drug rep's boyfriend spout off his knowledge of expensive wines. (What's the big deal about dead grapes?) I saw more of my attendings that night than I had for the entire previous month. I wasn't sure where they spent their hours at work. Clearly they trusted Corey, because they only ever rounded on the sickest of patients regularly and let Corey manage the rest (despite them being liable for every patient on the Green Team).

And the drug rep seemed like a real person, too. It must have been the fine wine. I was usually skeptical about a person whose job was to always be cheerful. I didn't care for actors, off screen. That's another reason I became a doctor, not a businessman.

Afterward, I kept thinking about Yoda telling Luke to beware of the Dark Side. I was sure I saw a glimpse of it. They really were trying to change me. Don't get personal with patients. Prescribe this drug. Doesn't the wine accent the filet well?

I'll never join you!

Chapter 15

Adios, Green Team. Hello, first of August. Eleven months to go. The first month had an extra week because we started the last week of June. This meant that the last month would be only three weeks long.

I joined the Subspecialty service. Urology, Neurosurgery, and Otolaryngology rolled into one. I could pick your brain, pick your nose, and—oh, never mind. Just a couple of interns and I worked directly with the attendings. We didn't have a chief to oversee us bumble our way through patient care. There should have been a public service announcement to warn people to stay away from the hospital.

Brodie, my partner in crime, if clean-shaven and nicely dressed, would have looked like the perfect Ivy League college boy. But he maintained himself pleasantly disheveled. His wavy blonde hair was just long enough to fall over itself in funny ways. And I don't know when he shaved, but it was never at a time that would allow him to look fresh for the hospital. I think his look was part of a master plan to create the illusion that he was always working so hectically, so devotedly, that he didn't take time out for grooming.

One of the anesthesiologists gave us some advice. "Call your attendings. Their goal is to never come to the hospital; they will abuse you. But remember, they get paid to staff these patients. Make them earn their money, especially when you don't know something."

Corey had said it numerous times, but in a different way. "Load the boat. Get as many people on board before it sinks, because if you're on alone there is only one person to blame. If you screw up because you were in over your head, it sticks on your record. You don't want that." When things were ugly with a dying patient, he would get the opinion of as many attendings he could. He would document the radiologist's opinion, the attending surgeon's thoughts, and his own in the chart. "CYA." Cover Your Ass.

The attorney put everyone who was involved with the patient's care on the initial list of people being sued. You had to work your way off.

I had no choice but to agree. I had zero training in neurosurgery and urology—not a single medical school rotation. I didn't have the experience, or the knowledge, to know when a patient should be rushed off to the OR for a craniotomy.

But that was fine. I had a whole day to become an expert. Brodie got stuck with the first night on call. Mine wasn't until the next day. I would have dreaded getting that first call, but Brodie shrugged it off. Anyone who could live in a tent on campus during college to not "waste" money on renting a place for a semester could handle one night of neurosurgery call.

Brodie answered our team's first page. "You want to go see some guy's penis with me?"

"Not really." I'd get my own consults in short time.

"That's too bad. The ER resident says it's really nasty. A paraplegic guy left his erectile aid on the last couple of days. He thinks we might have to cut it off."

"His penis or the erectile aid?"

"His penis."

"All right, I'll come." I'd never cut someone's penis off before. After gaining experience on toes, I was ready for the big time.

The ER room looked like the front cover of some never heard of rap album. The room was actually a normal, clean room. White linen on the beds, yellow tiled wall, bright fluorescent lighting. But smacked in the middle of the scene was a black man adorned in dark sunglasses with gold rims to match the gold necklaces piled up on his neck sitting in a wheel chair. A white sheet was draped over his lap. Two tightly clad women, one on each side of his wheelchair, fawned over him.

"Hi, I'm Dr. Roberts and this is Dr. Iaquinta. We're from the Urology service."

The patient waved the two women out of the room. They silently followed his orders. My first thought was He's a Pimp! A real live pimp.

You don't see them in rural Wisconsin.

He wasn't interested in pleasantries. "Just tell me I'm not going to lose my dick."

"What happened, sir?" Brodie excelled at calling everyone sir, just like Corey instructed.

Mr. Pimp explained he had used a penis pump to achieve erection and then he placed a rubber band at the base of his penis to maintain it. That was two days ago. He had forgotten to take the rubber band off after sex. He had reinserted his Foley catheter so he could urinate, but failed to notice the rubber band. Because he was paralyzed from the umbilicus (belly button) down, he didn't feel any pain.

Brodie removed the sheet. Most of the skin on his penis was dark blue and sloughing off. The stench reminded me of summer road kill, a few days old and maggot-eaten. One of those smells that can, and does, induce gagging.

Brodie and I just shrugged as if we had seen this a hundred times before. Brodie played his role to perfection. "You've got a bad infection, sir. You're going to need antibiotics. But I think we should get the plastic surgeon to see you, to get his opinion on the best way to treat you."

We covered up his diseased member and went out into the hallway. Brodie raised an eyebrow at me.

"You think he would have smelled it before now."

"The smell is probably what made him realize he forgot the rubber band."

"What are those two women still doing hanging around him?"

"I don't know. Maybe they're anosmic (don't have a sense of smell). They won't be around long if he lets them get a look at that thing."

We found the plastic surgeon, the same nice one who taught me about the sutures. Brodie's gruesome description inspired Dr. Thornton to come to the ER with us. I think he used the words "burnt, rotting Italian sausage."

The plastic surgeon's face fell when he saw Mr. Pimp's penis. I think he wanted to read the penis its last rites, but instead he reiterated that IV antibiotics were absolutely necessary.

Mr. Pimp sensed our lack of optimism. He tried to encourage our efforts. "I don't think I could go through the rest of my life dickless."

The plastic surgeon echoed that only antibiotics and a tincture of time would tell.

Outside the room Dr. Thornton told us, "If my pinky finger looked like that, I'd just cut it off."

I shuddered.

Maybe if he were a female surgeon he would have. But he understood. Removing a man's penis is likely to upset the Penis God. You never, ever, cut off another man's penis. You let it fall off on its own.

My urology experience continued. I left them to assist one of the urologists with a TURP (transurethral prostatic resection), which is the most polite way to say the urologist is going to drill a hole in just the right place to make a bigger passage for urine to flow. Old men who couldn't pee because their prostates were too large got TURPs. We inserted a rigid scope the diameter of a pen into the urethra. The end of the scope had a spinning blade on it. The urologist scraped away chunks of prostate and pulled them out of the penis. I squeezed my legs together so tightly that my testicles started to hurt.

The urologist had the build of a ZZ-Top guitarist. His fingers looked like bratwurst. They were too plump to be coordinated enough for anything but operating scopes. They were probably too thick to pick his nose, too.

Within minutes the urologist made it clear he was as disgruntled as everyone else. "This place makes me sick," he said. "I have to ask for everything I need here. Nothing is ever set up correctly. Nobody wants to work." He fidgeted with the scope and reinserted it into the man's penis with a speed that made a tear come to my eye.

"That's because they're all on salary," I said. "There's no incentive to work."

"I know. Sometimes I think I should quit practice and come here and run this place. The first thing I would do is fire everyone from the top on down. The administration here is as worthless as tits on a bull. You can't imagine how many millions of dollars are wasted a year."

"I'm getting an idea," I said. "I found out that none of our clinic patients are checked for insurance before seeing us. When we send them out for tests, x-rays, or CT scans, it is free until they are pre-opped (prepared for operation). But not everyone gets operated on, and some people get the operation denied because they don't have a payment plan. We are wasting hundreds of thousands just from clinic alone." I handed him another instrument while we chatted like two guys working on a car together. Instead, we stood trapped between a man's spread-eagle legs. But, you couldn't tell. Blue drapes covered everything except the man's penis.

"It doesn't stop there," the urologist continued. "I get paid for whatever procedure I bill the hospital for. But the hospital only charges the insurance companies for what is on the pre-op plan. Every time I do extra procedures I get paid, but the hospital has no system of checking. They aren't reimbursed from insurance companies. That's why they are always in the red." The suction tube filled up with bloody chunks as the blade whirled.

"If I were unethical I would have talked this guy into coming to my private clinic. He has Medicare. It would pay me more to have him come to my place and do the surgery there. He won't get billed for everything done here." He continued. "The hospital doesn't realize that these are sought-after patients. This guy didn't have to come here. Any hospital would have loved to have him as a patient; they'll get their money back."

Our next case was delayed because the room hadn't been turned over. The cleaning crew went on break just as we finished the last case. There are union laws that prevent the nurses from cleaning the room for the next case. (At least that's what the nurse told me.) In other words, a union law prevents a nurse from helping us get the job that needs to be done done. Another easy way down the path to the Dark Side.

Chapter 16

I started my first day of "subspecies" call delivering Corey's intravenous drug abuse speech.

We had debrided my patient's neck abscess, but you can only hack out so much dead tissue out of a neck before you hit a major vessel, important nerve, the airway, or the esophagus. Her neck looked like a mountain lion had given it a good chomp. So, I told her what we tell people in Old World County Hospital. I told her to shoot drugs into her leg and not her neck because we couldn't cut off her head when she got a really bad infection.

I said it with the same seriousness that Corey did, but deep down I didn't know whether to laugh or cry. In college, when people asked me what type of doctor I wanted to be, I never thought to reply, "The one who tells patients not to shoot drugs into their neck because we can't cut off their heads."

That evening I called Rachel to tell her all the crazy stuff. For instance, when I asked one of my neurosurgery patients how he was doing, he replied, "I want guns, knives, and alcohol." Interesting guy. Not the sort of hobbies I'd expect a computer programmer to have. But he wasn't quite himself after a blood vessel broke in his brain yesterday morning.

But the funniest thing I could come up with was that I was the in-house neurosurgeon on call for Alameda County.

She had her own amusing story about the dentist who lived down the block from her. He confronted her on her way home from the Med School and asked her out. She assured me I was safe unless she developed a cavity. We made plans for her to come visit in a few weeks. Then we played that game where she doesn't hang up until after I hang up. After obnoxious fake clicks I hung up for real, I needed some sleep. She never hangs up before I do.

A couple hours later my beeping pager startled me awake. Will I ever get used to that noise?

The digital readout said midnight but it felt later. I dialed the number without turning on the call room's light. Hopefully, I thought, it's nothing, and I can go right back asleep.

"This is Brad. Get down to the CT scanner. Now." Brad was the trauma chief. Not good.

I started my speed walk from the resident's call lounge down to the

CT scanner. What was down at the CT scanner? It had to be something lousy; why else would he have paged an intern?

I was sure that Brad didn't want me; he wanted my attending and needed me to call him. I jogged as fast as I dared in my wooden clogs. I tried to think of what I knew about neurosurgical emergencies, but nothing came to mind. Not because I was tired, but because I had never seen a neurosurgical emergency.

The trauma team stood huddled around the CT monitors like men in a bar watching the Superbowl on a four-inch television. I squeezed into the cramped quarters and closed the door behind me.

Brad looked over his shoulder at me. "Who's the neurosurgeon on call?"

"Blanchard."

He grunted. "Okay, call him. We'll tell you what to say." Blanchard had a reputation for not coming in while on call.

As I paged Dr. Blanchard, Brad presented the man in the scanner. He was forty-eight years old. He had been punched in the face in a bar, fallen back and hit the ground, knocked unconscious. He had come to by the time the ambulance had arrived. But when the paramedics escorted him to the hospital, he lost consciousness—an ominous sign.

"Yeah, what's going on?" Dr. Blanchard answered. Whenever I heard his Texas twang, I imagined a tobacco-chewing cowboy in worn jeans and boots. In person, he looked like an effeminate Englishman, small and dressed for an early afternoon picnic.

Brad flipped through the black-and-white images of the man's head on the computer screen. The CT scanner produces two-dimensional images of the head at different levels. In essence, it cuts you like a loaf of bread and we look at only one side of each slice. Brad started feeding me the "Magic Words" for Blanchard.

"There is a 48-year-old man who was hit and lost consciousness, came to, and lost it again en route," I said. "He is currently unresponsive and his CT scan shows a large subdural on the left with ventricular effacement and a two-centimeter midline shift. He is intubated and unresponsive." I was speaking quickly, because that made it sound more important. The Magic Words—effacement, midline shift, and unresponsive—meant the guy's brains were being squashed by the blood clot growing inside his skull.

"Take him down to the OR. Shave his head, start the case. I'll be there in a minute." Blanchard hung up.

Start the case? Just go cut open the patient's skull? Did he know to whom he was talking? I was suddenly in a movie—the wrong movie. I'm out of character. I'm supposed to be the jester. I don't know the script. What am I doing here?

I hit "O" on the phone.

"Hello, Operator 13," a woman answered.

"Hi. Can you tell me the pager number of the anesthesiologist on call?"

"There isn't one."

"What do you mean? There always is."

"Nobody reported in today and all the people we've paged say they aren't on call."

I hung up. The trauma team awaited my instructions. I didn't have any. I told them, "There's no one listed on call for anesthesia."

Everyone stood dumbfounded until they realized I was the naïf. There was always an anesthesiologist in house. I hadn't been here long enough to know it.

The other trauma resident, the unshakeable Asian woman, took command. "You bring the patient downstairs, I'll find an anesthesiologist." She said it with such authority I almost replied, "Sir, yes, sir."

Everyone split except for a nurse, the respiratory therapist, the patient, and me. We wheeled the patient downstairs. He didn't look like he had been punched. He looked like an ordinary guy sleeping on a gurney, except for the endotracheal tube coming out of his mouth. The respiratory therapist squeezed the bag at end of the tube to push some air into his lungs.

I grabbed a blue paper mask and hat as we wheeled by the shelves in the hallway. We got the gurney into the OR and the patient onto the table. The trauma resident had completed her mission; the anesthesiologist was waiting for us.

I put on the mask and hat. Blue-hatted, blue-masked people with white gloves filled the room. An outsider might think we were decontaminating nuclear waste, not trying to save a life. The patient was lying naked on the bed, his dark skin a stark contrast from the sterile whites and blues of the room. A nurse put compression stockings on his legs, funny we still worried about him getting clots in his legs when one was expanding in his skull.

The anesthesiologist hooked up all her monitors and threw a warm blanket over the patient. I grabbed a razor to shave his head. Dr. Blanchard strutted in. He had the blue hat and mask, but his scrubs were magenta.

"Can't do a case without the films, Sal." He grabbed the razor away from me.

"I'll get them." I ran off to the CT scanner. They weren't out of the printer yet when we left, but the excuse wouldn't have mattered to an attending.

When I came back, the head was shaved. Dr. Blanchard peeled open the patient's eyes and asked me for my flashlight. The pupils were fixed and dilated; no response to light.

"He's probably already dead, but let's go ahead anyway. Maybe we can salvage his organs." Blanchard's nonchalance must have meant he'd seen this a million times before.

What? I had thought we were going to save a life. If this was just about keeping organs alive, I might as well be sleeping. What if his family didn't want his organs donated? Weren't we supposed to believe he could still make it? Wasn't that why we're doing everything at top speed?

Blanchard went to scrub and I followed silently behind.

"What can I do to help?" I asked after we gowned and gloved.

"You can do the case," Dr. Blanchard said.

Nothing in his voice led me to believe he was kidding.

He drew a large, backward question mark on the shaved scalp. "Cut down to the skull on a ninety degree angle on this line."

"Knife," I called, and, unbelievably, the scrub tech put the knife in my open hand. I'm twenty-five years old and about to do a craniotomy. At this moment the moviegoers, sitting on the edge of their seats, feel a gnawing tension in their stomachs as they witness the knife being handed to the jester. The guy behind you mutters, "Nooooo." But it's too late.

I provided traction on the skin with my left hand and put the knife down. It sank through the skin like butter all the way down to the skull. I followed the smooth curve he had outlined.

"Slow down, it's not a race."

But this guy is dying.

He might already be brain dead.

When I finished, Blanchard pulled at the large skin flap I made. It separated easily from the pale skull. Everything turned red; the scalp really bleeds. He undermined the skin surrounding the wound and called for the hemo-clipper. The hemo-clipper looks like a Nerf toy made to shoot little banana clips.

"Just push in on the skin edge and click." When he pulled the trigger a little plastic clip, about one-quarter inch wide, shot forward and grabbed the skin edge, pinching the blood vessels closed. He handed me the clipper and away I went. Clip, clip, clip until the cartridge emptied, then a reload and more clipping. After about 20 clips, hemostasis was achieved.

"Great," he said as I finished. "Drill."

The scrub tech placed the drill into his outstretched hand.

"See this? It turns at 7000 rpm, so only put it on something you want it to go through. The pedal is by your foot." He looped the cord and wrapped it around my forearm and placed the drill in my hand.

I felt like a little kid again, playing with Dad's power tools for the first time. But the stakes were much higher.

He marked off four corners where I was supposed to make the holes. "As soon as you're through, stop. The goal is to not drill the brain."

This is all a dream. I'm not a brain surgeon. It's all make-believe. We're just playing doctor. It's the game of Operation.

I couldn't even see a body under all the drapes. I just had a square of skull with some blood. It could be fake. The only evidence of a live patient was the beeping of the anesthesiologist's heart monitor.

I hit the pedal and the drill whirled to life. It had its own mission: to skip across the smooth skull. But my determination prevailed—that, and brute strength. Once it bit, the drill sank into the skull. Dr. Blanchard kept the drilling area wet with saline. The saline lubricates and prevents dust and overheating, but it also causes splashing. I pulled up a few times to check my progress. I pulled up once more right as the resistance changed. I had created a clean, three-millimeter-wide hole into the skull.

"All right, you're doing great. Next hole."

I attacked the second mark. I didn't pull up as often. Dr. Blanchard was just about to say something when I pulled back. The second hole was done.

"Good," he said hesitantly. He decided to not admonish my speedy drilling.

After I made the other two holes, he called for the saw.

"If you hold it on just the right angle it will cut through the skull like air, otherwise it's work."

A saw in my inexperienced hand sounds risky, but it was actually one of the safer tools at my disposal. It has a guard on it that prevents it from going too deep.

"Connect the outsides of the holes."

Ho hum, just sawing the skull. I am sawing a human skull. I am sawing a living human's skull!

What do you do for a living?

I saw human skulls—live people only, of course.

Really? That must require a lot of training.

Well, I went to medical school for four years, but I don't remember any lectures about skull-sawing. In fact, I don't remember any neurosurgery lectures whatsoever.

How do you know what you are doing?

See the guy next to me? He's my mentor. When he's quiet, I can assume I'm doing things correctly.

But I didn't think I was. My angle must have been off, because my hand ached from trying to hold the saw in line.

When I finished, Dr. Blanchard took a small pick and lifted up the cut square of bone. It came right off. He set the bone in a sterile plastic container.

"That's what I like about these young skulls. They are so easy to open."

Hmm. I'd never had that thought.

The dura mater, a protective sheath just inside the skull—"dura" meaning tough and "mater" meaning mother—separated us from the brain. Blanchard poked a small hole in it with a scalpel.

"Take the scissors and cut out a flap."

"Scissors," I called. Tough mother? Hardly. It felt like I was cutting a mostaccioli noodle two minutes from being done.

We folded back the flap. I couldn't see the brain through the dark red clot. Again, I thought of food: It looked like cherry Jell-O.

"Be careful with that sucker. A neurosurgeon holds it like this," he ordered. He changed my grip.

"Never use full suction. It will suck up the clot and the brain with it."

I remembered reading that the human brain is the same color and consistency as vanilla custard. Fresh brains look nothing like the stage props in movies.

We started sucking away the clot with a coffee-stirrer-sized vacuum. I was glad they had machines for that. If they didn't, I would probably have to do it with my mouth, and that would be too disgusting.

We went through 1.5 centimeters of clot before we uncovered the brain's mysterious folds. I wished I could have taken a picture. There was something mesmerizing about the spider web of purple veins covering the pale yellow brain, almost like watching the pipes screensaver to see how it will cover the screen.

I find it hard to accept that something with such an ambiguous shape has so many functions. The brain is nothing like the stomach. You can look at the stomach and say the food comes in here and goes out there. The muscles jostle food and the glands secrete digestive chemicals. Straightforward and logical. The brain is just a squishy blob. You can't look at one wrinkle and deduce that the area controls leg movements. It would be easier to look at a record's grooves and guess what sounds are encoded.

"Brain retractor," Dr. Blanchard called. "If you use this, you can put your sucker right on top of it. Then you know you won't be sucking brain."

He slapped it into my hand. It was just a flat paddle of metal, like a steel tongue depressor. I slowly slid it under a clot slowly and sucked above it.

"Go ahead, you don't have to be so gentle. It's soft. It's a brain retractor." He politely omitted the "duh."

The room remained silent. The anesthesiologist, scrub tech, scrub nurse, and neurosurgeon were watching me suck away clot from the brain. If I suddenly went mad and started sucking up this man's brain, they would all witness it firsthand. Think of the stories they would tell!

"What are his chances of survival?" I asked.

"About one in five hundred."

So you're saying there's a chance. I manipulated a huge chunk of the clot onto the retractor and lifted it out. Just below the patient's head was a plastic bag, the Brain Bag, used to catch the dripping blood. I dumped the clot into it. Of course, some missed and splattered on my shoe. My mom would have a fit if she found out I forgot to put on shoe covers.

Fresh blood oozed out from under the edge of the remaining clot. I couldn't see the source. It kept bleeding and I kept sucking. Some dripped onto the floor, a bit more onto my shoes.

We flushed the brain with warm saline once I finished. The bleeding stopped. The brain was safe from being squished from another blood clot.

"Let's get out of here before the brain swells too large." If that happened, we wouldn't be able to put the bone back. Someone had accidentally thrown away the saved bone from the last guy Dr. Blanchard couldn't close. Dr. Blanchard wasn't too happy about that. The patient, of course, couldn't have cared less.

He let me sew the dura closed. After I did that with a baseball stitch, we put the chunk of skull back on. We attached little metal brackets to it to hold it in place. Those years of Erector sets paid off.

Dr. Blanchard inserted a long probe through one of the drill holes into the dura and one of the ventricles of the brain. This tapped the cerebrospinal fluid and allowed the extra fluid to drain as intracranial pressure increased from the swelling. We left the other holes open.

To close the deep layer of skin, Blanchard put in interrupted stitches and I tied them. We closed the outside layer with staples, which hold the skin together with greater strength than stitches. At least that's what the ER doctor told me in eighth grade when I had to get the back of my head stapled shut because the stitches kept popping.

Dr. Blanchard ditched me as soon as the patient left the table for the ICU. During the day, the ICU is an assault on your senses. Bright lights, foul odors, shrieking beeps, loud bells—I would go nuts if I worked there all day long. Thankfully, night was quiet and the lights were dim.

I found a cozy desk chair at the nurses' station and started writing the orders. I sat in a daze. I had just finished a case that fourth-year neurosurgical residents would have waited in line to do. I tried to focus on the task at hand; I had to figure out what orders I needed to write. A neurosurgical patient requires a fair amount of attention. The nurses have to keep an eye on anything that might increase intracranial pressure.

I dated and timed my orders. No wonder I couldn't think, it was 3:30 a.m. Out of the corner of my eye I saw someone walk out of my patient's room.

The woman, who looked about forty, was wearing a dark blue suit. It was an odd hour for business apparel. She spotted me amid the drab cabinets and counters of the nurse's station and approached me with eyes full of questions.

"Hello, I'm Dr. Iaquinta." I stood up and offered her my hand.

"Hi, I'm his sister, Tanya. Are you the doctor that did the surgery?"

"I'm one of them." No way I'd admit to full responsibility. I needed Dr. Blanchard to fall back on, in absentia. No family wants to look at an unshaven 25-year-old and imagine he just performed brain surgery on their loved one.

"How long before he wakes up?"

"He might not. He had a very severe bleed inside his head."

"But it was only one punch."

I cocked my head to the side. Was this denial? Maybe she's underestimating what one punch could do. More like just disbelief. I think of ninjas being able to kill with one punch, not guys in a bar.

She has to be his younger sister. Her skin is so smooth. She must be his younger sister.

Hello?

What?

Task on hand, the woman is waiting for you to answer.

Sheesh, sorry.

"It caused bleeding inside his skull. The brain cannot tolerate bleeding. It's like he suffered a stroke." I could have told her the Magic Words, but I suspected they would be meaningless to her.

"They arrested the guy who punched him."

89

I didn't know what to say. The only thing that I could think was that a single punch had probably made the guy a murderer. I wanted to be that blunt. Blunt seems logical. Blunt is efficient. But that wouldn't be the right way to convey her brother's dismal prognosis.

"What's that tube going into his head?" She asked. She certainly was calm; maybe because she was tired. It was the middle of the night.

"This is a shunt that allows extra fluid building up around the brain to drain." That one was easy to answer.

She left me to go into the room with her brother. I followed her for a couple of steps. He looked like the subject of an alien experiment. White blankets covered him up to the chin. An endotracheal tube protruded from his mouth, attached by a hose to the respirator. A second tube jutted out the top of his head and was attached to a pressure monitor. His eyes were closed and sweat glistened on his face.

Her eyes became glassy. "You better get better. Why are you always getting into trouble?" Her voice sounded more disappointed than sad. Maybe she was the responsible sister and he was the goof-off brother. She stepped forward to stand next to his bed. I backed up to the nurse's station to finish charting, and to give her some privacy.

Seconds later I heard the decisive click of her heels as she exited the ICU. I was surprised she didn't have more questions; maybe it was too much for her. As the ICU door closed, I realized my "Most Exciting Case" was her dying brother. While his family had been worried about him, I was thrilled to cut open his skull.

I'm a creep.

*

A couple of hours later my Adventures in Urology continued, as did one incredibly long shift. Yesterday made me happy to have a penis. Today made me insecure about mine. I thought I was doing all right in the size category (don't all men?) until I was called to the ER.

I hated walking into the ER. Patients in gurneys lined the hallway. They reached out toward me as if their hands were coming out of the walls in a horror movie.

"Doctorrrr," a woman moaned.

"I am not your doctor." I kept moving, too afraid to slow down because they might grab me and pull me in.

One wrinkled man had hair shooting out in every direction and eyes trying to bulge out of his skull to freedom. "My secret is going to come out," he chanted. "I can feel it." He looked straight at me, and I couldn't avert my eyes. "I can talk like this because I'm fuckin' psychotic."

Yes, you are. I rushed by, afraid his eyes would launch themselves at me. In mid-flight the pupils would blossom into mouths studded with small jagged teeth. Then, they would stick to me with a resounding plop and start devouring me.

They only put patients that required "high visibility" in the hallway—the very people that should be tucked away into a dark corner. One of those psych patients had given a medical student the experience of a lifetime a few days earlier. One of the ER's frequent flyers complained of abdominal cramping as usual, so the attending sent a medical student to do a history and physical on her. The astute student noticed her large abdomen but the patient adamantly denied being pregnant. She "just had a big stomach." However, when it came time for the exam she had a foot sticking out of her vagina. The whole way down to the OR she continued to scream that she was not pregnant. Would everyone stop asking me that?

I walked into Room 12, where a young black man fidgeted in his seat. "Doc, you've got to help me. You've got to do something. I can't get rid of my hard-on. It hurts." He didn't look like my usual early morning patient. Most of them were people that were finishing a long night, whereas he looked ready to leave for work in his crisp khakis and thin blue sweater.

I wanted to tell him that an erection was nothing to complain about and that there were thousands of men that would love to be in his pants (sorry about the pun)—but he didn't seem in the joking mood. So, I held back and went for the double entendre.

"How long has it been?"

"Two days. My girlfriend gave me a blowjob and it never went down."

"Were you using any devices?" If you say a rubber band I'm going to pass out.

"No."

"Are you on any medicines?"

"No."

"Take any drugs?"

"No."

"Do you have any other health problems?"

"No."

"And after you orgasmed it stayed hard and hasn't gone down for the last two days?"

"Yeah, look."

I could see by the bulge in his khakis that I wasn't dealing with a teeny weenie. He unzipped and withdrew a county-fair ribbon-winning zucchini from his pants. Cripes, there is an elephant in your trousers!

His engorged member flopped onto his thigh. I winced at the taut skin; a single pinprick and it would explode like a water balloon.

I immediately took the necessary first step. I excused myself to page Brodie. I had to return the other day's favor.

A few minutes later Brodie bounced into the ER. We tried everything to get Mr. Hard-on flaccid—phenylephrine, terbutaline, nude pictures of Roseanne Barr—but nothing worked. I suggested we submerge his genitalia in ice water, but Mr. Hard-on declined. Just the thought would make me flaccid.

In the meantime we sent his urine for a drug screen as well as for infection. Infection was unlikely, but drug use was still a possibility. He looked like a clean-cut guy, but you know the rule: Trust no one.

"We've tried a lot of things, sir, and nothing has worked. We could stick a needle in it and drain the blood out." Brodie offered. I shot Brodie a skeptical glance.

"Fine. Do anything. Just get it down." Mr. Hanks' desperation convinced me that Brodie's plan might be the only thing we could do.

When Brodie stuck in the needle, it didn't pop. And sure enough, 40 milliliters of blood sucked through a 22-gauge needle made him flaccid.

His urine tested positive for cocaine. He lied to me. I like how a patient can lie to doctors without consequence, but it would be unethical, even grounds for a lawsuit, for a physician to lie to a patient. Maybe he didn't know that patient confidentiality prevented me from reporting his drug use to the authorities.

"Your urine test came back positive for cocaine."

He didn't even pretend to look sheepish. "Yeah, I use it sometimes."

"Did you use it the day you got this erection?"

"Yes."

"Do you want to tell me exactly what happened?" This was like pulling teeth. Actually pulling teeth is easier, you just rock them back and forth with pliers and out they come. Little did I realize back then, but I think my dad got his jollies from having kids shed their deciduous teeth. He pulled all my loose ones.

"I injected some cocaine into my penis because I heard it gives you a better erection."

Oh! You injected cocaine into your penis! Did that little tidbit escape your mind when I asked you what happened earlier? Or when I asked if you used drugs? Is cocaine not a drug anymore? Do you realize you are putting yourself at risk by not telling me there is cocaine in your system? You're the guy who makes us say the patient "denies" drug use.

"Oh. You shouldn't do that; you'll destroy the blood vessels in your penis." All those things I wanted to say weren't really necessary. Well, most of them. "You should have just told us at the beginning. We need to know what's in your system; it might interact with some of the drugs we give. We don't tell the police. Do you need help quitting cocaine?"

Offering him assistance psychologically relieves the guilt I'd have about sending this guy back to the streets. I didn't expect him to say yes.

"No, I rarely use it."

"Well, then don't use it at all."

93

Chapter 17

My "cranie" (craniotomy) patient from the other night didn't respond when I pulled his eyelids open. I shined my flashlight into his eyes but his asymmetric pupils didn't constrict. He didn't blink when I touched his cornea. I pinched his skin with my fingers. I squeezed the tip of his index finger as hard as I could between my thumb and stethoscope edge. I rubbed a knuckle firmly on his ribs. I put all my weight behind it. Not a single response.

I wiggled his endotracheal tube. He gagged weakly.

Not brain dead. Yet.

I dreaded meeting with his family. How was I, a neophyte, supposed to talk to them about their dying loved one?

"What do you expect to happen from here?" Tanya, his well-dressed sister, asked.

"I don't expect much. There is almost no chance that he will ever regain any function." I struggled to tell them the blunt truth. And lying was out of the question; there's no point in it.

They tried to maintain their composure as I delivered the bad news. But why try? If there was any time to lose composure, it was right then. Why insist on acting tough? Someday a giant meteorite will crash into the earth and kill everything. The last ten Americans will stand around with their hands in their pockets like nothing happened, saying, "Yep, I'm okay."

His mother gave me a pleading look. His wife distracted herself by looking into the corners of the room. Tanya remained serious.

"What do we do now?" She wanted the bottom line.

"We wait and see. In a couple of days we will know how things are going. It's too early to tell." The majority of patients in this scenario will die within the first five days. "This is a time where you pray." If I hadn't seen mom with a Bible earlier I wouldn't have said that in our overly politically correct, hypersensitive world.

"But, this is also the time when you should figure out what he would want." I instructed. They all looked at me quizzically.

"I was in the same situation with my father," I said. "He once told me that if he would never be able to go golfing or fishing, he would not want measures taken to keep him alive." My eyes started to get wet. Measures taken. Sheesh, I really was turning into a doctor. "You have to think about what he would want, not what you would want, and that is the most difficult thing." If I blinked, a tear was going to fall from each eye. They could lose composure, but their doctor couldn't. It didn't matter; they could see it in my eyes. They all had the capacity to pity me in their time of grief. They must have been good people.

Tanya saved me from talking. "So, all we can do is wait and see?"

"Unfortunately, yes. I wish I could tell you everything will be okay, but I can't."

"We'll see what the man up there has planned." Tanya looked up.

"Yes, the frustrating thing is that we are always last to know." I turned to the mother and put my hand on the side of her shoulder. "I'm sorry."

"Thank you."

I didn't have to say anything else. I turned and walked away. The mother's look had said thank you louder than her voice ever could. I knew she appreciated my honesty. I did a thousand times more good with that conversation than I had done the other night in the operating room.

This was the hard stuff in medicine that no amount of schooling could teach. It comforted me to know that I could do it. Maybe it was just in me, or maybe it was the experience of my father's hospitalization that gave me the ability to sympathize with them. Or maybe it's because I haven't been anesthetized from seeing this a hundred times.

*

The fog never lifted on Saturday, which suited me just fine. If it's gloomy, I don't mind being trapped indoors. People stay in on dark days instead of crashing their cars or falling off their ladders while cleaning the gutters. They don't even bother shooting one another. Nobody likes getting their guns wet. If next weekend is nice, Brodie's going to regret switching calls with me.

The time of year was the second factor that kept people out of the ER. In the fall, all of the rabble-rousers stayed home and watched football. Head traumas wouldn't occur until after the game when they were too drunk to walk, or just drunk enough to beat each other silly.

A quiet call day tempts you to do something. If you fully devote your attention to anything, like reading a book, you will get paged. They know. If you go grab breakfast, they know. They even know right when

95

you've loaded up your tray and are standing in line waiting to pay. Then they page and it goes off like a fire truck's siren. And because you've put the ceramic cereal bowl on the right side of the tray you can't let go with your right hand to silence the pager; so you struggle with your wimpy left hand. And because you aren't immediately silencing your pager everyone else begins trying to balance their tray on their knee to check their own pager. And when you finally hit the button on your pager the return number is just "3," a mis-key. Which means you will wait for eternity for the second page with the correct extension.

But, I believed in karma. If I did hospital work, I would not be paged. If I surfed the Internet, a train wreck would arrive. But if I went into the hospital to check on all my patients, nobody would come. So, I rounded slowly on the weekend. Spent some time with the patients.

Most of my patients were neurosurgery nightmares. People in the worst of situations...for the most part, comatose. I still said hi to them. And checked them like a gardener checking his roses.

Len Leigh, my one communicative patient, always greeted me with "Hey, Doc." He said it in a long drawn-out way that made me imagine he was still stoned from his hippie days. His long black beard and scraggly hair supported the image. Of course, his back pain required copious amounts of narcotics, which further supplemented his personality. He was only 47 years old and already failed chemo for a kidney cancer that invaded his spine. He chose for us to reinforce his vertebral column with a spinal fusion. Then, he wanted to live the rest of his life with only palliative care. I didn't chat long because his girlfriend had arrived.

After making it through the rest of the day and night without a single call, my pager awoke me at 6:30 a.m. Only one-half hour before Brodie relieved me! My fifty-hour shift was almost over!

I returned the page.

"Hello, Doctor?" It was one of the nurses. "I am calling about your patient, Mr. Leigh. His respiratory rate is only six a minute." The normal rate is twelve to fifteen breaths per minute.

"How is he oxygenating?"

"We didn't measure. But he has a mask on." She sounded defensive.

Great, a mask. What good does that do if he isn't actually inhaling?

"Is he arousable?"

96

"Wait a second," she replied. I could hear her ask another nurse, "Is he arousable?"

"Not really, he seems really tired."

"I'll be right there."

It sounded like a morphine overdose. Opioids suppress the respiratory drive; he could suffocate to death.

I started for the door when I realized my bladder needed immediate attention. I couldn't hold it all the way to his floor. I ran to the bathroom.

Emptying the bladder is a "primitive" reflex. A full bladder signals the spinal cord to loosen the sphincters so it can drain. This does not require thought. Your brain learns to suppress the urge until you are at a socially acceptable receptacle. You can toilet train, but you can't toilet rule. You cannot decide to hold your urine for two days; your bladder reflex will win. I learned my limits while scrubbing in on a ten-hour liver transplant.

I envisioned myself in court trying to explain why I went to the bathroom. The defense attorney would ask me if I ever heard of the marathon runners that wet themselves while running the race. Well then, Dr. Iaquinta, isn't your patient's respiratory status more important than a simple footrace? Your selfish devotion to your bladder is NEGLIGENCE!

With fists pounding on the wood railing, the jury would start chanting. GUILTY! GUILTY! GUILTY!

I finally finished. I ran down the hall and down the stairs and to the next building. I had to get up to the seventh floor. The good news was that the hospital had four speedy elevators in the central area. But the bad news was that two were out of commission. In addition, the sanitation experts had a habit of cleaning elevators at inopportune times. A balding man lazily waxing the elevator floor looked at me like I was an alien. Wait, I was an alien—I'm not from this planet.

I sprinted up the stairwell and burst into the hallway out of breath. I took a few deep breaths so that I could act like I didn't just leap up the stairwell. I don't know why.

I rushed into Mr. Leigh's room and flipped on the light. "Mr. Leigh?"

He didn't stir. An oxygen mask sat perched over his mouth. I inspected it, waiting for it to fog up as he exhaled.

One. Two. Three seconds.

Nothing yet. There are usually four or five seconds between breaths.

Four. Five. Six.

The nurse said he was breathing slowly.

Seven.

Eight.

Come on.

Nine.

Ten seconds.

Why wasn't anyone in the room with him?

Eleven.

Jesus, man, breathe! Nobody dies on my shift unless it's planned!

Twelve.

I reached for my stethoscope. I noticed the CODE button on the wall.

Thirteen.

I bent down toward him. Breathe!

FOG! The masked steamed up with exhalation. Whew.

I looked at my watch. It took another fifteen seconds for him to expire again.

"Mr. Leigh, wake up," I barked into his ear.

His eyes crept open but drifted closed within seconds. He looked like the kid in a teen flick that smokes too much weed. He looked like everyone else on my service: unresponsive.

"Len! Wake up. How are you?" I hollered, giving him a shake.

"Enhhhhhhhh," he moaned.

It's alive! Alive!

His eyelids wiggled, but were too heavy to open.

I ran down to the nurses' station because no one had come to help.

"Who is taking care of Mr. Leigh?" More accurately, who's not taking care of Mr. Leigh? "I need 20 milligrams of Naloxone, now." I wasn't in the mood for please and thank-you. Why was he alone when I got there? Why did I have to leave him alone to get the antidote?

A chunky nurse plodded over to the medication cabinet. She retrieved some vials and handed them to me. Then, she meandered into the supply room to get a syringe. She didn't seem to sense my urgency.

"Why don't you come with me to administer this?" I asked.

"No, I don't even think I can give that."

"Sure you can. It's up here on the floor."

She claimed she was too busy and started fiddling with some supplies.

Okay, I'll ask here. "Why was Mr. Leigh alone when I got to his room?"

"What?" She said, digging through a drawer of syringes. I could see that the roots of her blonde hair were dark.

"Why was he alone?"

"I have other work to do." I wanted to spank her fat butt. If there ever was a time someone deserved a spanking, it was now.

"You called me concerned about his respiratory rate. If you are worried about someone's breathing, then you should stay with him until help arrives. Who's going to hit the "code" button if you are out here?"

"This isn't the ICU. I have other things to do. We don't sit with patients here."

Forget spanking, she needed to be throttled. But I didn't think I could get my hands around her thick neck.

"If you don't think a patient is breathing adequately, you can't leave him alone."

The other nurses at the station watched. Some nodded in agreement. The others thought I was a bothersome jerk.

"I have other patients to manage." She turned away.

Was I speaking her language? She has no clue what I'm getting at. One of the times you leave a patient like him alone, he will die before the doctor arrives. What would you call his condition if he were breathing four less times a minute, like say zero times a minute?

I wanted to grab her shoulders and shake her and scream, "What would you do if that was your son in there? Would you just walk away?"

There are only a few basic rules in life. Remember what my mom said? Even Dr. Fagan said it. Treat other people the way you would want them to treat you. If I'm breathing four times a minute I don't want anyone deserting me in the hopes that a doctor will come by soon. But, if I yelled at her then I would be breaking the rule.

"Just give me the syringe." I snatched it from her hand and marched down the hall. I didn't have time to set her straight. As it was, I committed the same crime by running down the hall to get the Naloxone—even if it was only 30 seconds. I tried to convince myself that she didn't know the mistake she made by leaving him alone for five minutes. The alternative was abominable. It couldn't be true. Could it?

I went into Mr. Leigh's room and administered the Naloxone. In a few minutes his breathing rate picked up to normal. He woke up.

"Good morning. How are you?"

"Good, how are you?" He looked over at me, undoubtedly wondering why I was sitting in his room. He hesitantly brushed his snarled hair away from his eyes.

"I'm fine. Do you remember me coming in here a few minutes ago and trying to wake you up?"

"I think so," he said with a puzzled look.

"I think you had too much morphine last night. To put it in lay terms, I think you were stoned out of this world."

"Ohhhhhhh." I expected him to follow up with a "cool."

"I am going to hold some of your pain meds this morning. If you start having pain, ask your nurse for them."

"Sure. I'm fine now."

"All right, I'll see you later." I looked at my watch. I had about twenty minutes before the Naloxone wore off. Not a single nurse had stopped by while I was in with Mr. Leigh.

I told his nurse that she might have to administer more Naloxone. She checked her watch and silently confirmed she'd be leaving soon, too. I knew I couldn't trust her to check on him every five minutes.

I wrote the appropriate orders to transfer him to the ICU, where a nurse would actually watch him and administer meds. Then I documented what happened in the chart. I omitted the apathetic nurse from the story because it seemed wrong to write about her in the patient's chart. I didn't even fill out a complaint about her, because of what the urologist said, bad employees get promoted because firing is impossible.

Brodie paged me from the call room. I met up with him and signed out.

Fifty hours straight at the hospital topped off by a nurse trying to kill my patient. If I could manage that, they couldn't break me. Sure, I might turn into a bitter jerk, but they wouldn't break me.

After that week, I felt I could go and do anything in life. Maybe not be an actor or concert pianist, but most other things would probably seem easy in comparison.

Maybe I was getting cocky. Maybe I was just learning what I was capable of when pushed. Maybe this was why they waited to give us real white coats. They needed to see who would stick around for it.

Chapter 18

We finally got our real white coats—our nameless loaners were replaced by coats with our names embroidered onto them. When I pulled the crisp, clean coat over my blue scrubs, I felt like a real doctor. Now I could find Franklin and strut proudly past him.

Wait. What's this? My name isn't embroidered onto the coat. It's embroidered on a patch that is ironed onto the coat. This thing could just rip off. Nope, they don't expect permanence.

Those fools. I'd never quit. I bought a set of oils just to see if I could paint. And I was there for the same reason. I loved challenge. I wallowed in adversity. You try to kill my patient? Your inadequate healthcare won't break me. You give me a lousy iron-on nametag to rub in how temporary I am? HA! I'm going to superglue it on. Don't you know I never give in? You'll never stop me!

Cripes, I needed sleep.

Chapter 19

The fifty-hour shift paid off. The following Friday, Brodie let me out early as an extra favor. Rachel arrived that evening for her first visit since I started residency.

As soon as we got to my apartment it became obvious that I needed her around. Who else would inform me that normal people didn't change shirts four times before ending up in the same slouchy T-shirt and jeans before going out to dinner? She commented that I was more of a girl than she was.

And I was "anal" about the way I loaded the dishwasher. Anal? No, highly efficient. Waste was sinful. Okay, it wasn't sinful. I don't have religious motivations for any of my actions. But somewhere there must be a tiny god who smiled every time he saw me cram the dishwasher as full as humanly possible before running it.

Every little thing she nitpicked about meant that she noticed me. Dr. Fagan didn't even know the color of my hair, but Rachel noticed everything. And Rachel had positive energy. She lived at a level of happiness significantly above mine. A faint smile always rested on her lips, like she was still remembering the punch line of a dirty joke. Hopefully, she'd never become a surgery resident.

That night, after our late dinner, Rachel put on a pair of my scrub bottoms as we got ready to go to bed.

"What are you doing?" I didn't like the hospital reminder, but at least they were clean.

"These are comfortable," she replied.

I looked at her and said, "I don't want no scrubs."

She laughed.

The rest is private.

Chapter 20

When I returned that Monday I found an elderly white man lying in place of my "cranie" patient. My patient had died over the weekend, and just as Dr. Blanchard had hoped, they decided to donate his organs. At least something good came out of the tragedy.

The paraplegic man with the rotting penis returned to the ER that morning. This time he came alone. No girls. No penis. He still had the Foley catheter entering the blackened head of his penis. The majority of the penile shaft had rotted away, leaving the catheter visible as it entered a pus-covered stub protruding from his pubic hair. A thin bridge of tissue rested on top of the catheter and connected the groin mass to the necrotic head. I knew that if we took out the catheter the rest of his penis would fall off.

"Oh, my dick. My dick's gone." He cried. "What can I do? What can you do?"

"We need to wait until the infection is gone. Then, we can discuss possible reconstruction options." I wanted to cry, too.

I looked again, mesmerized. Calling Brodie would only insult our patient. Only one option remained for the poor guy. He needed reconstruction for both the physical and psychological benefits. I couldn't imagine the county approving the numerous necessary operations. If we couldn't operate on all the people with gallstones, how could we get him into the OR to rebuild a penis?

I didn't know what to say to a man who had lost his penis.

Everything will be okay.

That's a lie!

How horrible for you. We'll do what we can.

You're darn right it's horrible.

At least you have your health.

FUCK YOU!

I patted him lightly on the shoulder. It could have meant whatever he wanted it to. He didn't mind. He looked at me and shook his head slowly.

These moments of futility were worse than everything else put together. Why can't I be omnipotent?

I wished I could rewind two days and be hiking with Rachel in

104

Point Reyes. We had a leisurely walk through nature out to the beach without so much as a thought about rotting penises. Someday the world will be full of robots that can do all the work and humans will have nothing to do except watch movies and go on hikes. That's why Rachel's visit was so great; we were living in that future for a weekend.

But now I know why soldiers aren't granted leave during war. Once in battle mode, it's best to stay in it.

I came across another intern, Kendra, as I walked back toward the ICU. Normally, when I pass a fellow resident I give him or her nod of acknowledgement. There's seldom time for more. That, and I'm closemouthed.

She forced out a "Good morning."

She was clearly fighting her own battle. First of all, it wasn't morning. Second, she had her scrub top untucked. Dr. Organ warned us not to "dress like the janitors." Her stethoscope hung onto her coat pocket for dear life. Kendra usually looked discombobulated, but not distressed. She had the bloodshot eyes of someone who cried all night long.

"What's up?"

"I'll tell you in just a minute, just let me finish this. You're going to hear about it anyway so you might as well hear it from me." Her high voice cracked. I expected a break down.

Did she get fired? Did she quit?

I followed her down the hallway. She stopped and turned toward me, and the dam blew open. "This morning I was scrubbed in with Dr. Irving on a trauma. I was holding back the intestines as she tried to control some bleeding near the kidneys when she asked for a vascular clamp. So I got one and handed it to her." Kendra looked up and down the hall. "She grabbed the clamp from me and whacked my arm with it, hard. She told me that it wasn't my job to hand her instruments, it was the scrub tech's." Tears built up in the corner of her eyes.

"I can't believe that." Dr. Irving didn't really do that, did she? We weren't on the East Coast and this wasn't 1960.

"I know. I was in shock. I was like 'whoa, you just hit me.' I just got hit. I didn't even say anything. Nobody did, the scrub nurse, the circulator, and the anesthesiologist were all silent.

"And my arm hurt," she continued. "But I couldn't move it. I had to hold the guts out of the way." Kendra put her stethoscope into her pocket and straightened her coat.

"Man, I think I would've left. I don't think I could have kept standing there."

"I didn't want to let her win. I just sat there in silence. I held the intestines for over an hour. Nobody said anything the whole time. I was seething. But then I started hiccupping."

A few people walked past us in the hallway. She waited for them to get out of earshot.

"Dr. Irving looked up at me and said, 'If you can't control yourself you can scrub out.' I told her I had the hiccups, but she thought I was sobbing. That made me angrier. My hand froze from retracting so long. I couldn't even move it after the case. Then, I wasted the rest of my morning going to the ER to document everything."

"I can't believe she did that. She must have some good lawyers in her family."

"I know. I totally wish I could press charges. I don't even know what I should do."

"I don't know either." The higher-ups were Dr. Irving's coworkers. And they were the same attendings that controlled Kendra's future.

"The rest of my team told me to forget about it. And now they are avoiding me on top of it, like I did something wrong and shamed the team. I can't just forget about it. Do you tell a woman to just keep quiet about domestic abuse?"

"No, but if you make a complaint it could be held against you. These people write the ticket to where you go next year." She was a transitional intern; she was only here for a year before going on to another program. But she didn't have that program arranged yet.

"I know, it sucks. But this is bullshit. I was thinking about staying here, but if this is how it is, then forget it." She looked at her pager. "I've got to get out of here, but if you have any good ideas let me know." She stormed off.

Program directors liked things to run smoothly. I could guess Dr. Organ's twisted logic. It's okay if physical abuse got swept under the carpet, just as long no one knocked on his door to bother him about it. He'd probably have a cutesy little saying like, "Nothing bad happens to a

106

good intern."

Then he'd remind Kendra how much worse residency was when he went through it. He survived as a black man progressing through a pyramid program fifty years ago. Ten interns became eight second-years to six third, four fourths, and then two chiefs. The abuses they inflicted on one another to get ahead had to be worse.

Dr. Organ called a meeting with all of the interns that afternoon.

As we filed into the conference room I remembered what Corey once said: "If God were an elderly black man he would look just like Dr. Organ." Dr. Organ sat at the head of the table waiting for us. The evening sun came through the picture windows behind him and outlined his tall, lean frame. It lit up his silvery white hair, which glowed against his dark skin. He had his head held up with his eyebrows a little raised so that he was looking down at us as we walked in. He looked like a skeptical God watching the humans down on earth. It looked like he knew the answers and he was curiously watching us fumble our way toward them. Of course, this usually was the situation.

He was all-powerful. If he was quiet, the entire room was quiet. And if someone dared talk, a single glance would strike him mute.

He waited until we all took our seats. He looked us over and smiled. "I'm impressed by your Musketeer attitude. It's great that you could all take time out of your busy schedules to come to this meeting to show support.

"You've formed a cohesive group early in the year. You can use this. You will find good working relationships are absolutely necessary to practice medicine," he segued. "The better rapport you have with ancillary staff, the easier it will be to do things that are right for your patient but not necessarily by the rules."

What about Kendra being hit? Nobody said anything. Dr. Organ charmed us with more compliments. Kendra sat dumbfounded. Suddenly, Dr. Organ was saying, "What a beautiful evening. You should all go and enjoy it. Incidents happen, but I'll take care of everything." And with a wave of his magic wand he herded us out the door.

We filed out of his office like a bunch of confused cattle too bewildered and too scared to moo. He called after us, "Anytime you have a problem, feel free to stop by. Enjoy the rest of the day."

On the way out, Kendra muttered, "That was pointless." Everyone nodded in silent agreement.

His promise to "take care of things" did not mean that he would take care of them in a way that wasn't detrimental to Kendra. It might have been a "take care of things" in the Mafia sense. Where was his loyalty? To his staff, or to what was right?

*

My alien anthropologist voice kicked in. On my planet we didn't have physical abuse. We used to. But, after years of scientific study it was determined that it was an inadequate form of communication. Ironically, rather than get the person to do what you wanted them to do, it actually alienated them from you. I suspected that in time all humans, too, would learn that lesson.

*

I didn't get to enjoy the evening. Instead I found myself in the ICU for a couple hours, facing the distraught husband and son of a stroke victim.

Making diagnoses had become easier with practice; I memorized drug information effortlessly and I quickly learned and absorbed treatment strategies for disease. But I struggled with delivering bad news. As a youngster, I knew I wanted to be a doctor. I knew what wounds looked like, because I split open my knee in fourth grade. When we dissected frogs in eighth grade, I imagined operating on people. But I never imagined looking into an elderly Asian man's eyes and telling him and his son, a son who looked a few years older than I was, that his wife was unlikely to have any meaningful recovery from her stroke.

"But how do you know, Doctor?"

Good question. Because of my vast experience? No, because of Dr. Blanchard's vast experience and everything I've read on the subject.

"I can't say with absolute certainty. It takes a few days to tell. But, when we see a stroke like this, the prognosis is bleak." I pulled out her CT scans and pointed out the damage; this allowed them to see something wrong. Until that moment, "Mom" just looked asleep, but now she had a visible problem. Reviewing the scan also averted their eyes from mine.

I pointed to the white blotches throughout the brain. "This light gray tissue is normal brain. All the bright white spots are blood in the brain. Getting blood on the brain is like dumping jelly inside a computer. Everything short-circuits." That was the line the doctor told me as he reviewed my dad's CT scan.

In this case, the white blotches dominated numerous cuts of the scan. She didn't have a little stroke; she had Old Faithful.

I recommended that they talk together about the quality of life that she would want. A couple weeks of neurosurgery and I had that speech down pat. As they stared pale-faced at me, I noticed how much the son looked like his dad. Not the time to joke about how the apple didn't fall far from the tree.

As I walked away I wished that they could somehow know how much I sympathized for them. How could that woman's husband look at me, one-third his age, and expect that my sympathy was genuine?

Chapter 21

A year ago, I had awakened to the phone ringing. It was 5:30 am. Despite having two other roommates, I knew it was for me. I was the only one who got called that early. It was always bad news. My sister's suicide attempt had been a 5:30 am call.

"Your dad is on the way to the hospital in the ambulance." It was Kim, my dad's girlfriend. "He got up to use the bathroom and he took a few steps and stumbled to the floor. He started slurring his speech and couldn't move. He's unconscious. The paramedics just left."

"All right, where did they take him?"

"To Memorial; I'm going there right now."

"Okay, call me as soon as you get there and let me know what is going on."

*

I immediately picked up the phone and called my older, more reachable, sister, Lisa. I told her the limited information I had and it was all that she needed to get her moving. When the situation is serious, my sister can snap to attention and take action. No doubt she flew out the door before the phone settled back in its cradle.

After I hung up with her I continued to get ready, without the urgency I imagined Lisa had. I lived hours from the action. Nothing I did right now could matter. I live in Logic. Emotion is a small town nearby; I only pass through it now and then.

The only thought I had was that my father was going to die.

I didn't bother waking up my roommates. I had my Rice Chex for breakfast like usual and the phone rang again. It was Lisa.

"Hey, Dad had to be intubated and they are going to transfer him to the neurosurgical unit at Froedtert in Milwaukee. He'll be there in about a half-hour."

Lisa often starts sentences with "Hey" as if she needs to get everyone's attention. She had already called mom and planned on meeting her at the hospital, and she agreed to call Jill.

"Drive carefully, no sense speeding here." Lisa knew Logic too. She could be cold like surgical steel when needed and she could give a look to cut right through you, something that if I tried I'd start giggling if you didn't laugh at me first.

110

I packed an overnight bag and then I went to my medical school's hospital and met up with my team. Mind you, I was a responsible medical student and I didn't have the phone number of a single person on my team. I have this stupid sense of dedication to anything I'm part of, such that even in times of calamity I adhere to the plan. Maybe I should have been a soldier.

After watching the residents divvy up the day's work, I pulled the chief aside. I shocked him with the latest update on my dad. He looked flabbergasted. I felt like I just told him that it was his dad that was in the ICU. I'm sure he thought I had a bad relationship with my dad because I came to the hospital instead of hitting the road as soon as possible. I didn't bother explaining my sick sense of loyalty to my job, even if that job is meritless and nearly meaningless. As a medical student I was the bottommost part of the totem pole...the part buried underground. If I looked up I'd see the intern's soles.

As a fourth year medical student, even without the neurosurgery rotation, I knew rushing to Milwaukee wouldn't make a difference. Intubating someone after a stroke is a terrible prognostic indicator.

Then everything became surreal, like I lived underwater. I flowed out to my car. I put a CD in the player and started off toward Milwaukee. I'm surprised I can't remember what CD I listened to; inane details often get etched into my mind. I still remember what song I was listening to when I got my only speeding ticket four years ago.

I only had one thought the entire drive. My dad had a stroke. My dad had a stroke. My dad had a stroke.

Seventy-five minutes later I walked into the Neurosurgical ICU and spotted my dad lying in bed, with the back raised. A white tube stuck out of the top of his head. It looked like a science fiction gadget the aliens use to steal memories. Instead it was the same intracranial pressure monitor and shunt that I'd put in less than a year later on a man punched in a bar.

His face puffed out like he had an allergic reaction. Even his eyelids were puffy. His face looked naked without his glasses. I could count on one hand the number of times I had seen my dad without his glasses. He would even swim in our pond wearing them.

A second tube protruded out of his mouth. Apparently the aliens also took interest in his throat. The tube ran to a respirator that sounded like a compressor. It delivered slow breaths, like Darth Vader.

An IV stuck out of his right neck and another in his right arm. The sheet was pulled up around him. Crisp and white. If they pulled it up any further I'd have thought he was on the way to the morgue.

He sat perfectly still. Then I noticed my older sister draped over a chair. She told me they had to put "that thing" in his skull because the pressure in his head was too high. Mom was down in the cafeteria. Jill and her husband, Jeff, weren't there yet. Every conversation I'd had with Lisa started like a news debriefing. She was my right hand man bringing me up to speed before the big meeting.

She told me that the doctors had called it a hemorrhagic stroke. She pointed to two men in white coats across the ICU.

The Neuro ICU was a horseshoe of 10 rooms around a large nurses station. Every room had small groups of distraught families huddled together. The two doctors were examining films on a view box. As I approached them, I guessed that they were looking at my dad's films. Of course, anyone in the Neuro unit could have had a giant stroke.

The older one, an Indian man, turned to me and said, "Hello." The other one looked only a few years older than I was. I presumed the older one was the attending and the younger was his resident. Both men struck me as peaceful.

"Hello, I'm Sal." Lisa would have already filled them in about me.

"Hi, I am Dr. Patel and this is Dr. Anderson," Dr. Patel introduced. "Your sister tells us that you are in the last year of medical school."

"Yes, not much left now." I didn't want to facilitate the small talk.

"What are you going into?"

"ENT," I replied, looking at the scans over his shoulder. I could see lots of white.

"Oh, that's a great field." He either just finished establishing rapport or he noticed me inspecting the scan behind him. "We were just looking at the CT scan."

"Wow," I remarked flatly. The right hemisphere and the basal ganglia were lit up. The midline of the brain was shifted left. The brain's swelling had pushed the ventricles closed. All the Magic Words to get a neurosurgeon's attention, except that the clot was in the brain, not on it.

"Your father had quite a serious bleed," Dr. Patel confirmed.

"What sort of long-term resolution do you see with something this bad?"

112

"It isn't good. You can see blood throughout the basal ganglia, internal capsule, and into the right hemisphere. In addition, his brain stem has been compressed, resulting in the need for intubation." Goodbye motor function. The best-case scenario would still leave his left side paralyzed.

I appreciated that he spoke to me like a physician. I didn't want to hear anything but the naked truth doctors give each other out of earshot from the families.

"Was it an aneurysm?" Why else should a 51-year-old have a stroke? Give me more than bad luck.

"We haven't found any evidence of one."

"Is it worthwhile to continue care?"

"I usually recommend waiting five days before withdrawing care. If the miracles are going to happen, they happen in the first five days." He pulled the films off the view box.

My education prevented me from having false hopes. I didn't plead, "Is there anything you can do?"

"I can talk to you about what is going on and you can explain it to your family, but I think some things will best be heard from my mouth."

That sounded good. You be the bad guy, just in case any of my family members want to kill the messenger.

I went back to the room. "Hi Dad, how are you doing? If you wanted to hang out with me today you could have just told me last night."

Lisa looked up and smiled.

"How are you doing?" I asked her. Her eyelids were puffy too.

She told me that Mark, her husband, had a case with a surgeon in the same hospital that day, and he'd be back up soon. Mark worked as a sales rep for a surgical instrument company.

I looked at my dad for a while, then touched his right hand; his left hand probably had no feeling. I half expected the skin to be cold. It was discomforting to touch his hand and feel its warmth when he seemed so dead.

Jill and her husband arrived shortly later. Jill seemed remarkably calm; maybe the shock of the situation made her somewhat withdrawn. I noticed her shirt had long sleeves that covered the back of her hands.

Those sleeves always created the question, is she hiding the past or the present? The accumulated damage from needles never disappears.

Later that afternoon, when my sisters, their husbands, and my mom were there, the neurosurgeons talked with us. They explained that my dad had had a "very serious stroke." They said that his condition was like opening up a computer and throwing jelly into it. If it worked at all, everything would likely be garbled. I liked the analogy enough that I filed it into my long-term memory not knowing it would have future use.

They suggested that we think about what my father would have wanted as a quality of life. They recommended we wait five days before making any decisions just to see if any sort of progress would be made. In lieu of a neurosurgery rotation in medical school, I was getting firsthand teaching.

I went back to my apartment that night. I didn't see any reason to deprive myself of sleeping in my bed. I didn't expect any change at the hospital. Besides, Lisa had decided that she was going to stay at his bedside.

When I returned to my apartment I got out my brushes and acrylics, sat at the kitchen table, and started painting. I began my favorite backdrop: a blue sky that fades from bright blue at the horizon to midnight blue at the top of the canvas. I go back and forth across the canvas a few hundred times so that the gradations and brushstrokes are invisible. I candidly informed my roommate of the situation. I remember him saying, "You're going to be a great doctor. I don't know how you can sit there and just go on. You remain so calm."

"I don't know if that's so admirable. Some people might think that I don't care. Sometimes I wish I could break down just to know what it's like."

I don't know what was wrong with me. I was numb. Nothing ever felt like it was really happening to me. I ran into this over and over. Rachel didn't believe how important she was to me because I was never ecstatic around her. It wasn't her. I was never ecstatic. When I went whitewater rafting the guide said he wanted whatever drug I took because he never saw someone so sedate through Class V rapids. Everything was just another thing.

The next morning I went to the medical school library and found a few articles on the prognostic indicators of long-term survival after a stroke. One article said that one-half of the people in my father's situation would die within the first five days. Another 25% would die soon afterward and most of the remaining would remain in a persistent vegetative state. About one in five hundred would have some return of function. Nowhere did it say that there were patients who recovered the ability to fish or golf.

The other papers were just as grim.

*

I went back to Froedtert. There hadn't been any change.

I said good morning to my dad and then examined him closely. His pupils didn't react to light. I inconspicuously squeezed his fingertip between my finger and a pen; he didn't withdraw from pain. I wasn't surprised.

I hadn't been surprised all along. His girlfriend's phone call hadn't shocked me. The evening before the stroke occurred I had had a premonition. I was in my dad's car approaching my apartment when it happened. I thought that something bad was going to happen in the family. I specifically thought that my dad was going to die. That surprised me because I didn't think that he would be the first to go of the five of us given Jill's recent history.

Ever since that moment, the events seemed to be following that path. And I merely watched the movie. Maybe that explains why I was so calm. If we all followed a path chosen by karma, or whatever, then extrinsic events didn't have any weight. Then my father's death became the equivalent of driving to the grocery store. People aren't full of emotions while driving to the grocery store, right?

My mom stuck around that whole day. It might have seemed odd, given that my parents had finalized their divorce the week before. But I could see that she still cared. She also said that she was around for us kids, especially me, because I didn't have anyone else, whereas both of my sisters had their husbands. I appreciated her company.

Friends and relatives stopped by all day, even people I didn't know. They all recognized me. When I was created, my father's genes beat my mother's to a pulp. One time a hairdresser told me I looked just like my dad did when he was my age. She then went on to tell me how she had such a crush on him back then. I never went back to her again.

Everyone looked to me for information because I was the medical student. I didn't want that role; I just wanted to be the son. But I knew the answers to most of their questions, and I was available.

115

My great aunt disapproved of me considering withdrawing my dad's care. One of her sons had died young, and she had encouraged every possible measure to be taken to prevent his death. But I knew what my dad wanted. And dealing with my aunt's disappointed attitude once or twice a year would be easier to handle than the guilt I would have if I didn't follow my dad's wishes.

By the fifth day, nothing had changed. My sisters and mother supported withdrawing care. They knew that my dad would have been wanted to be able to fish, balance his checkbook, and feed himself. These didn't look like possibilities given that he couldn't even breathe on his own.

The whole family—his aunts (even the one with silent disapproval), uncles, cousins, and us, came to say goodbye that evening.

They let me go in first to say goodbye alone. It was strange how that happened. I didn't ask to go; they just said they would wait for me.

During the past few days, I had become head of the family. My great aunts and uncles started to treat me like they had treated my dad. My dad's employees informed me that if anything ever happened to him, I was in charge. It had been the same way when his father had died. As far as I knew we weren't part of the Mafia, but everyone sure acted like it.

I went into the room alone. "Dad, I am sorry it had to be like this. You know that I love you. You were a best friend to me. I am going to miss you." It was redundant to verbalize it because I knew he knew it already. "If you are in there and can give me a sign, now is the time. Just wiggle a foot or an eyelid." I stood quietly watching. I shook my head back and forth slowly. I didn't cry; I hadn't even shed a tear about the situation. I felt guilty. What was wrong with me?

I gave his thumb a pinch, just to see if he would wiggle, but he didn't. I waited another minute and went back to the waiting room. The others then filed down the hall. I sat alone for a moment when my little sister ran back into the room.

"Dad just opened his eyes!"

"What?"

"He opened his eyes!"

I jumped up and ran down the hall. Everyone was ecstatic. My great aunt kept repeating, "We love you, Sam," over and over. I could see that his right eye was opened more than his left and he even moved his right foot. I ran over to his side.

"I'm here, Dad," I exclaimed. When I took his right hand he gave me a light squeeze. "This is a miracle!"

"We were all in here saying goodbye and he wasn't moving or anything, but then when my mom spoke he moved," my second cousin said. "Her voice woke him up."

"I was in here not ten minutes ago and he didn't respond at all."

Everyone stirred around the bed, telling my dad how much they loved him. After the excitement calmed down, I asked him some questions.

"Dad, squeeze my hand twice if you can understand me," I commanded. He gave me two squeezes. I couldn't believe he was conscious.

Everyone watched me, waiting for my questions.

"Dad, I will ask you yes and no questions. Give me one squeeze for yes and two for no, okay?" I asked.

One squeeze.

"You had a bad stroke five days ago. You have had us quite worried. Do you understand?"

One squeeze.

His right hand let go and weakly crept to his left chest. He touched it like someone feeling an object in a bag trying to guess what it is.

"Can you move your left hand?"

There was no movement. The half of his face that could move wrinkled with frustration.

His right hand came back down to mine.

"Can you feel on your left side?"

Two squeezes.

"Could I have a few moments alone with my dad?" I asked everyone. They all nodded in agreement and left the room.

My dad made a writing motion.

"You want to write?" I inquired. "Sure, let me get you something." I grabbed the nurse's clipboard at the bedside, a pen, and a piece of paper. I put the pen in his hand and held the board underneath it.

He held the pen and wrote. I could not discern a single letter from the scribble he made. I suggested he tried to write one letter at a time.

Nothing changed. It was a scribble.

"I can't read that, Dad. Is the first letter an A? B? C?" I asked. At "I" he tapped.

"I love you?" I asked.

He gave me a thumbs-up.

"I know that, Dad. I love you, too." I knew he knew it. In fact I had told him so on the phone, the night before he had his stroke.

He tried to write. It hurt me to see him so incapable. He gave up. I had the suspicion that he thought he was writing normally, but then he figured out that the inability to write was one of his many deficits.

I asked him a few questions and told him I would let the others talk with him and that I would be back. He gave me a squeeze.

My sisters went in one at a time to talk to him. This was the "just five minutes" everyone wishes they could get. Both were on bad terms with him before the stroke and they were able to make amends. I knew that the week before, my dad had tried to apologize to both of them about the walls between them. My older sister had turned him down for lunch after he apologized to her. That was the last she had spoken to him. I had seen that eating away at her over the past five days. I think that is why she stayed at the hospital 24/7; it was her own marathon of penance. If he was going to come to, she was going to be there.

Then, my mom went in to make peace with the man she had been married to for 29 years. He, too, had called her and apologized within the past week. He had told her that even though things hadn't worked out between them, she had done a great job as a mother. That meant a lot to her; he had blamed her for Jill's heroin addiction, a strike below the belt during an argument months earlier. She had carried that on her shoulders for months.

How did he know to make amends? Why this last week when the problems had been going on for years? And if it was something he sensed, then maybe I sensed it too?

*

Two years earlier, my parents had announced they were going to divorce. This wasn't a big surprise. Six years before the announcement, my mom and little sister had moved to my grandfather's house when we were remodeling our house, and after the house was finished they never moved back.

At first, I told my parents that I wouldn't choose sides and they promised that they would keep us kids out of it. However, as things progressed, it became apparent that my dad had done more wrong than my mom. He had blatantly lied to her and tried to hide assets from her. Worst of all, he had been dating his "new" girlfriend for approximately four years.

It disgusted me that he could be so dishonest. My parents had raised me to tell the truth. They doled out punishments to us kids when we'd lie. I had avoided deceit and the man I was trying to impress had turned out to be a liar. And as I witnessed the consequences of his lies, I vowed to always be honest. I could no longer see the point in lying. Maybe I should have thanked him for teaching me what not to do.

As the truths became apparent, my sisters cut him out of their lives. My little sister occasionally called him to ask for money, but after a while he got sick of it. Once the money stopped, she didn't call anymore.

I became the only person in the family that he talked to. Both his parents were deceased, and his daughters were on our mother's side.

*

After everyone had gone in to say goodbye, the rest of the family and I reconvened in his room. I took control of the conversation. I didn't know how long this moment of lucidity would last.

"Dad, I have some serious questions to ask you."

One squeeze.

"Do you remember the conversations that we had about your quality of life if something like this ever happened?"

One squeeze.

"Do you want to go through rehabilitation?"

Two squeezes.

Everyone was watching.

"Dad, do you want us to continue support?"

Two squeezes.

I had to be sure.

"Dad, do you want the machines stopped?"

One squeeze.

"Dad, do you realize that if the machines were stopped you will die?"

One squeeze.

He understood what he had asked for. But I had to ask the ultimate question for my relative's sake.

"Dad, do you want to live?"

Two squeezes.

Every face in the room grew long. They had all witnessed the boss of the family make his decision. He absolved me of all responsibility for his outcome. It was a small relief, given the gravity of the situation.

"Dad, when would you like us to stop treatment? Tomorrow?" I asked.

Two squeezes.

"A few days?" I asked.

Two squeezes.

"Later tonight?"

Two squeezes.

"Right now?"

One squeeze.

That squeeze crushed my heart. How could he want to stop now? We were having a conversation. Couldn't he at least wait a few days? We could have hours of conversation. I had so many questions to ask. I wasn't ready to take over his responsibilities. I wasn't ready to say goodbye now that he was awake.

"I love you, dad."

"We all love you, Sam," my great aunt said. A chorus of I-love-yous followed.

My dad gave me one last squeeze and withdrew his hand. He didn't move.

I went out in the hallway and told the nurse that my father had chosen to stop treatment. It pained me to honor his request while he could still communicate, but as it was he never stirred again.

I walked away from my dad's room with my mom when it struck

me. My number one fan had just deserted me. I stumbled to the wall and crumbled to the floor in the hallway. I started sobbing violently. I could hardly breathe through my tears. My mother reached her arms around me to cradle me.

I couldn't stop. I gasped for air between choking sobs. Then my mom started crying, too. She cried for me; my pain hurt her. She hadn't seen me cry since I was a little boy. And instantly I became her little boy again, crying in her arms. And for that moment she was mom more than friend.

After five minutes everything stopped. The two of us sat on the floor in a nook of an empty hospital hallway and talked. I can't remember what we said. But, from that moment on, nothing else seemed to hurt; it would all be so minor in comparison.

He didn't even have normal reflexes the next morning.

My dad didn't stir for three days. He had long shallow breaths, each one seeming like his last. My older sister, mom, second cousin, and I sat in that room all day long and told each other stories; sometimes about my dad, sometimes to my dad. We actually enjoyed ourselves. We had accepted that my dad had died three days before, when he had stopped communicating.

On the third day, I excused myself from the group to heat up some food in the microwave at the nurse's station. As I got up to walk out of the room, I took a long look at my Dad. I went over by his bed and touched his hand. I almost said this out loud. Dad, I am going to get some food. I want you to come with me. But when I come back, I don't want you to come back. Okay? Let's go get food. It was perfectly logical; my dad loved food. I should have said it out loud. My family wouldn't have thought much of it. And, it would have made it legitimate.

It took me about five minutes to heat up a plate of leftover Chinese food. As I walked back to the room the nurse was coming out. "I think your dad just took his last breath. Your family thought you might want to stay in the hall a minute before going in."

My family knew I was apprehensive about seeing my Dad die. I don't want my last memory of anyone to be the moment of his death. I avoid funerals for that reason too; memories of living people are more fun. But once again, nature miraculously worked in my favor. It wasn't a minute later when my sister opened the door to the room and peeked out toward me.

Nobody cried. We were all sad, but the mood was one of relief. The suffering had ended.

Chapter 22

So, I knew what it meant to receive the news I gave that man and his son. And maybe it wasn't important that they knew that I could sympathize. Maybe they just needed what Dr. Patel and his resident gave me: peaceful and patient delivery of horrible news, a chance to answer my questions, and a meeting with the family to reiterate the news and answer their questions.

That next morning, the woman still remained in an unresponsive coma. I flopped into a chair at the nurse's station to write my note when a strange odor invaded my nose. The odor didn't belong in a hospital and I immediately suspected my other patient down the hall.

The nurses began squawking like upset chickens. "Do you smell that?" "Is that smoke?" "Is someone smoking?" "Whew, you smell that?"

They all started poking their noses around like lab mice.

"Mister Pine! You can't smoke in here!"

I smiled. I wanted to stick up for Mr. Pine. He was a dialysis-dependent diabetic, and not a candidate for a kidney transplant. He also suffered bilateral above-the-knee amputations, heart disease, and he took enough pain meds to put down a horse. If anyone deserved a cigarette, he did.

I caught Evan grinning from across the station. He enjoyed seeing the nurses ruffled up. He slapped shut the chart he was holding and motioned with his head toward the stairwell. I tossed my chart onto the rack and followed him. We had a couple minutes before our M&M (Morbidity and Mortality) conference.

"My son took his first steps yesterday." Evan grinned.

"That's awesome."

"Yeah, but I was here."

"Sorry."

"Yeah, my wife paged me to tell me. But he was asleep by the time I got home." Evan shook his head.

When we signed in at the front table of the conference room I noticed that the list of patients to discuss were in a pile under Dr. Organ's arm. Usually we'd each grab a paper off that stack so we could read the summaries of every case to be discussed. When I turned to sit down I noticed an unfamiliar man and woman in the back of the room.

I sat down. A few more people filed in and took their chairs. Then Dr. Organ looked directly at the well-dressed couple. "Please introduce yourself and tell us why you are joining us this morning."

It wasn't an invitation; it was an order.

A short, black physician stood up. He approached the podium, adjusted his glasses, and straightened his white coat. Coats that crisp and clean don't take care of patients. He had just lost any chance of earning respect from this crowd.

"Good morning, I'm Dr. Nison. I'm here to explain why we are having an RN come to your M&M conference. She is assigned to look for sentinel events. These are events that could have been avoided and will be avoided with further training. She will look for these events so that they can be pointed out to the faculty. This way everyone will learn how to avoid making mistakes."

A sentinel event in the medical world is any unplanned occurrence that leads to patient injury or death. A simple example would be operating on the wrong ankle. The RN intruder worked for a committee that tried to find errors, or potential errors, and then create failsafe mechanisms to help prevent them. For example, creating a system whereby the operating surgeon and nurses confirm the site of the surgery with each other and the patient before sedating the patient.

The administrative doctor continued, "These events will be discussed by the appropriate committee. Then, the appropriate staff will be taught how to avoid such errors. This staff could be nursing, anesthesia, or surgeons."

Wow, a bureaucrat. I'm so glad that I avoided politics and pursued medicine. It only took a few minutes of him talking in lazy circles and generalizations before I felt like jamming knitting needles into my ears.

"How is an RN supposed to listen to surgeons and decipher which events need reporting?" the doodling trauma surgeon asked. Then, turning to the RN, "No offense to you."

"She doesn't have to make that decision. She just needs to report anything she might think is a sentinel event to our committee. Then the situation will be examined."

"Excuse me," Dr. Blanchard interrupted. Despite not being around much on call, he did come in for M&M conference. His patients comprised the bulk of the first "M," Morbidity. "This woman is an RN and you are going to have her sit in on our meeting? Wouldn't she be best used elsewhere in the hospital? I can't even get an RN on staff in my clinic and you are going to pay someone with her level of training to sit in a meeting? That's just wrong."

"We feel that this is the best way to use her services. Every time she picks up on an event that can teach a lesson to the hospital staff, she will be affecting many lives. The incident will never happen again."

I remembered what the urologist said about administrators. They were promoted to the position because they couldn't be fired for being lousy workers. My respect for the intruders started circling the drain.

Dr. Nison, Doctor-Adminstrator, obviously didn't know the content and format of our meetings. The faculty didn't sit around and blame ancillary staff for what went wrong with a case. The faculty sat around and blamed the residents. We talked about the case, the outcome, and what would have made the result better. We could spend a half hour discussing the different surgical options for a case in which the patient went home perfectly healthy.

"Why don't you just have us report the sentinel events to your committee?"

"You are supposed to. When JCAHO (Joint Commission on Accreditation of Healthcare Organizations) came here, they criticized the lack of reporting we had. We had only six events reported last year. The number should be much higher than that."

JCAHO is the committee that inspects hospitals. They measure the quality of care at each facility and compare it to the standard of care. They also check compliance with health care laws. It was a well-known fact that the hospital had performed unfavorably in the recent review. There were also theories that the people who worked for JCAHO actually had no concept of what healthcare was, and that they were forever reinventing forms, documenting procedures, and words to keep themselves in business. The signs in the OR were replaced with signs that had Braille in order to comply with new rules—at a cost of greater than ten dollars per sign. But I'm sure it was well worth it, because after that the blind surgeons didn't walk into the wrong room.

Dr. Blanchard's Texan twang picked up a notch. "Okay, we did lousy with JCAHO, but just answer these questions for me. Who is more qualified to diagnose a case of appendicitis, a board certified surgeon or an RN?"

"The surgeon."

"And who is better qualified to perform an appendectomy? The board certified surgeon or the RN?" Blanchard continued.

"The surgeon, but…" Dr. Nison started. He knew where Blanchard was leading him.

"NO, just let me finish here," Blanchard interrupted. "Who is better to discuss the case and determine if there were any extenuating circumstances, or sentinel events, that have altered the progression of the case? A room full of board-certified surgeons, or an RN?"

The administrator wouldn't give Dr. Blanchard the satisfaction of answering his question. "She needs to stay," he said.

"We would be happy to provide you with a list on a weekly basis of anything that might be a sentinel event. You've never even asked us." Dr. Irving, the trauma surgeon that hit Kendra, was now getting into the argument.

"Yes, I have. Dr. Organ has been aware that all cases that might involve a sentinel event should be reported. For two years we have only six cases. Second, she is trained to look for sentinel events."

"Well, these last two weeks were the first many of us ever heard of sentinel event reporting," Irving continued.

"That's not my fault."

"Why don't you just give us a chance to report these events?" Irving pleaded.

Suddenly the very people responsible for turning us into mature surgeons started whining like little brats who weren't getting their way. Any moment now Dr. Irving would probably leap out of her chair to whack the administrative doctor with a clamp she kept holstered on her hip.

"What other service in the hospital has a weekly conference to discuss every case that happened that week? None of them do, so why do you have to come here?" Dr. Organ asked.

"Medicine has an M&M conference," Nison answered.

"How often?" Dr. Organ asked.

"Once a month."

"And how many patients does the medicine service admit on a weekly basis?" Dr. Organ asked. Didn't this man see the trap he was falling into?

"About 80."

"You're telling me that once a month the medicine service has a conference and they discuss 360 cases? I don't think they do." Dr. Organ argued. "This conference is a tradition dating back a hundred years. It has always been closed to everyone except surgeons. This is where we pick cases apart and scrutinize each other in attempt to make ourselves better surgeons. This has nothing to do with the rest of the hospital. We don't talk about what we thought was anesthesia's fault or what was a nurse's fault."

"I still think this would be the best way to pick up sentinel events from a surgery standpoint."

Dr. Organ wouldn't have it. To anyone else's ears M&M would have sounded like a lawyer's cornucopia, not because there were so many botch jobs, but because the American public believed "complication" meant a botched job. Our society expected perfection from physicians. The public didn't understand the true complexity of a case. Two people could be diagnosed with appendicitis and both would expect the same outcome: remove it and go home. But what the surgeon found upon opening the abdomen could make a 25-minute case into a two-hour case. When that happened, we talked about what made it a two-hour case and why didn't we know it beforehand.

Regrettably, some wounds would get infected. Sometimes neighboring nerves, muscles, or organs would be damaged during a procedure. M&M focused on what might have been missed and what could be improved. We all wanted to learn how to be perfect; most surgeons deserve credit for trying to get performance to match their ego.

Dr. Organ stood up. "This morning's conference is canceled. Everyone is excused. We will reconvene at a later date." Dr. Organ paused and looked directly at the residents. "I feel sorry for all of you going to practice surgery in this time. You have none of the control but all of the responsibility."

Everyone sat still for a moment. Slowly, people stood and left, exchanging glances. Evan and I shrugged at each other.

The administrator didn't argue.

Chapter 23

The next morning we held a secret M&M conference at 6 a.m.

Dr. Organ started it with, "The last thing I am going to have is some nurse pass judgment on me."

Kendra rolled her eyes. She had confided in me the day before that she "didn't like surgery enough to deal with all this ego bullshit and the long hours. I want to be able to enjoy life." She was looking into family medicine residency programs, preferably somewhere with good weather. I couldn't argue otherwise. Surgery isn't one of those things you talk someone into. If you can't see the carrot in front of your nose, no one can show it to you. The big glorious carrot of working slightly less hours after you finish residency, but now assuming the full responsibility of your patient's care, being mentor-less in the OR, and all the paperwork to yourself.

You have to really want to cut people.

*

It was the first day of my third month. I had made it through the first two months without killing any of my patients and without any of the staff killing me. As my third Herculean task, I had to survive one month on Dr. Organ's team. I looked forward to operating with him. What type of surgeon was he? Was he a nitpicker? An instrument grabber? A case stealer? A laidback joker? (I doubted that last one.)

We started with the re-repair of a perforated duodenal ulcer. Right now, anything our patient swallowed leaked into his abdomen through the hole in his intestine. After the previous repair the surgeons left a drain next to the ulcer that exited out of the skin of the belly. Like a bad magic trick, when he drank blue-dyed water it came out of the drain.

Dr. Organ proved to be consistently inconsistent in all regards. He barely let Corey perform the operation. He constantly grumbled that Corey wasn't reading his mind. But he said it like, "I wanted you to cut that first before you tied this." All of his advice was after the fact unless it was a direct order. Cut here. Tie that. Just Bovie through it.

At the same time, he maintained conversation during the entire case, mostly complaining about the equipment for his own entertainment. "Normally, you wouldn't use these scissors for this, but these are County Steel. In a real hospital these would cut right through any tissue and you wouldn't want to dull them on suture. But here, they are barely sharp enough to cut a stitch."

I laughed politely.

Then he'd change personalities. "Corey, are you trying to sabotage this operation? This is supposed to be abdominal surgery, not abominable surgery."

Then he turned to me, "Sorry for raising my voice."

I watched Corey's every move. He didn't look like a botch artist to me. He made every move, every cut, deliberately. I felt like I was watching my sister put the final cards on a giant house with the anticipation of destroying the structure. I fought the urge to dig both my hands into the patient, and squish everything around. Then I'd say, "Well, thanks for having me. I really must be going now, have a good evening," and stroll out of the room.

Dr. Organ interrupted my daydreams to give me his Common Things are Common lecture. He delivered it regularly during conferences, but that didn't stop him.

"Dr. Iaquinta, I always guess the common disease because I'll be right most of the time; you can guess the rare disease and you will rarely be right." I nodded as if the information caused a revelation.

He refrained from telling me about perforated ulcers. He looked at Corey. "Nice move. That's how you should dissect." Then he looked at me and said, "I better be careful. Complimenting him is like pouring kerosene on fire."

He used unpredictability as a tool to keep the residents scared of him. If the underlings stayed confused, they couldn't organize a revolt. He must have read the Art of War.

Halfway through the case Dr. Organ said it was time to close. I thought the statement was just another weird joke.

Corey thought so too. "But we haven't fixed the duodenal perforation yet, sir." Corey never failed to call him sir. A stellar resident.

"Corey, I'm not even going to worry about that thing. It's fine. Look, there's no leak." He pointed to the visible part of the duodenum.

"Sir, we gave the patient methylene blue to drink. Not long after it showed up in his drainage bag. That drain sat right next to his previous ulcer repair."

"Enough of that nonsense," Organ barked. "We're done here. I am not going to go messing with that. You're just wasting time. Here, look."

He exposed the part of the duodenum that had the previous repair. He dumped a basin of warm saline into the abdomen, submerging the duodenum.

"Push some air down the NG." Dr. Organ ordered the anesthetist. The anesthetist grabbed an empty syringe and attached it to the nasogastric tube.

No air bubbled up from the previous suture line.

"See, no leak. Now stop acting ridiculous and close this up." He stepped back from the table. "Iaquinta, come around and help close. Remember, it doesn't take two hours to close the abdomen. Thank you, everybody." With that Dr. Organ ripped his gown off and walked out of the room like an actor strutting offstage.

"Ohhh, he frustrates me," Corey said. "His ego gets in the way of correctly finishing a case."

"So, are we going to fix that leak?"

We brought the patient to the OR to fix that leak. I didn't want to round on him every morning and watch him stagnate up on the seventh floor knowing that we didn't finish the case. And, I definitely didn't want to have to tell him a week from now that he required another operation.

"We'll try to do something," Corey replied. "Look, if he walks back in, thank me for showing you the portal anatomy."

"Huh?"

"Sometimes he walks back in," Corey said hastily. "I don't want him to know I am trying to fix this." He reached into the patient and exposed the previous ulceration. He called for a stitch and tacked down the tissue. Dr. Palm Pilot's stock on the Iaquinta Exchange soared with that bold move.

We continued to close. I think the average general surgeon looks at closing like doing the dishes; a lousy job that would ideally be done by someone else. But I like closing. I like the idea of putting everything back together. It's tidy. That's one of the reasons I'm going into ENT. Cutting things out of people's faces requires you to be sneaky; it's a game of   How-Big-of-a-Surgery-Can-I-Do-and-Leave-No-Evidence-of-it-Behind.

Corey let me sew the layers of the peritoneum and the abdominal muscles back together. We use such large needles, and only millimeters away from the bowel. What if I had this weird seizure and my arm jerked up and down stabbing the bowels with the needle repeatedly? It could happen any second now.

"Hey, I heard about Kendra getting hit," Corey said, interrupting my daydream.

"Yeah?"

"I also heard from Dr. Irving the interns were coerced into meeting with Dr. Organ to stick up for Kendra."

"What!"

"Yeah, man."

"Why would she say that?"

"I think she got it from an intern with his own agenda."

Corey confirmed my first suspicion. Shady Man. The doctor that looked too old to be an intern. The shifty guy. The only other guy without a Palm Pilot. Shady Man was a transitional intern, here for a year unless they offer him a position to stay. A weak attempt to ingratiate himself. Idiot. The Dark Path is easier, not stronger.

So much for unity.

By the end of the day I felt like I was in high school. Some of the interns circulated a sheet of paper stating that we weren't coerced into supporting Kendra. They wanted me to sign it. I didn't understand the point; it still didn't change the fact that she got her arm whacked.

Everyone except Shady Man signed it.

Chapter 24

Dr. Organ continued the secret 6 a.m. M&M conferences to avoid the administrators. All patients needed to be seen before conference by Corey. We had eight patients on service and Corey wanted to round at 5:20 a.m. I went to bed at 8:00 the night before so I could get to the hospital by 4:20 a.m. I had to write a note on all of the patients before Corey saw them.

On average, I spent ten minutes per patient. That included finding their chart and vitals. The progress notes and vitals flow sheet are often kept in two separate charts. Between the nurses and the gremlins, those charts were never together. Then, I checked the labs on a patient. The computers were the newest things in the hospital and had been quite advanced when purchased about twenty-five years ago.

I didn't get the results of half of the labs I had ordered the night before. The orders simply vanished overnight...repeatedly. I transcribed the results of the successful labs into the patient's progress note and onto a list I carried with me. Even if the chart disappeared between the time I wrote the note and Corey saw the patient, I had the results ready. As for the missed labs, I took the blame for those.

Then, we'd see the patients. How are you doing compared to yesterday? Better? Worse? Or, the same? Any nausea or vomiting? Are you passing gas, having bowel movements? Is the pain controlled? Did you get up and walk?

Corey taught me about the surgical "triple point," a.k.a the xyphoid process. This is the bottom of the rib cage in the center of the chest. It is highly inaccurate, but lets you know that the heart, lungs, and bowel are all making noise. Just once I'd like to pull the stethoscope away and say, "Hmm. Your heart just stopped. I give you about ten seconds."

When Corey arrived, we ran from room to room. Outside the door I briefed him on how the patient felt, the vitals, pertinent physical exam, and lab results, and what I thought we should do that day. We only reexamined the patients I thought had deteriorated from the day before. While we rounded we inherited a patient from the Medicine service. We were told she had diffuse abdominal pain and fevers, but the other docs didn't have any labs or films yet. We hoped to have some answers after conference.

*

After our secret M&M conference, I bumped into Dr. Organ in the hallway. "Iaquinta, what service are you on?"

"Yours, sir."

"Good," he said, "keep up the good work."

I wondered if he had Alzheimer's disease. We had been working together for the last two weeks, and he didn't remember that I was on his service. And yet, he had incredible recall of articles that were twenty-five years old. There were only two possibilities: I was not important enough to commit to memory, or, he couldn't form new ones.

But you wouldn't expect someone with Alzheimer's to be so amazingly functional. When Corey presented the new patient that we took on our service from the Medicine team, he insisted on seeing her. Corey warned him that we didn't have any results back, but Dr. Organ waved him off.

I watched Dr. Organ evaluate the patient from the moment he entered the room. The woman sat upright in bed, taking shallow, quick breaths. Beads of sweat glistened on her forehead. Dr. Organ knew she was in distress without even touching her.

Corey started to tell him which labs were pending.

Dr. Organ dismissed any further information. "We need to get this woman down to the OR right now." Corey sprang into action faster than he could say "yes sir."

When Dr. Organ wants to take a patient to the OR there are suddenly more people willing to help than I knew even worked in the hospital. A moment later we were in the operating room slicing open her abdomen. Brownish white pus rushed out at us.

"Dr. Organ, how did you know we needed to bring her to the OR right away?"

"By her exam."

But you didn't exam her. Not with your hands.

"Don't they teach you the history and physical exam in medical school anymore," he asked, "or are you all just high priests of the laboratory? You do plan on using the history and physical when you go into practice, don't you?"

"I'm learning."

"You young doctors believe that laboratory values and radiographic studies make decisions. Don't fall prey to how the ER manages patients.

I know that they get a CT scan before they call you. The art of surgery is being able to make a clinical diagnosis.

"If you're just going to look at the labs and the films, you might as well sit at home in front of your computer. They can just beam you the information and you can make your diagnosis without ever seeing the patient."

All right, you made your point. But in all of your jesting, you failed to teach me how you determined to take her to the OR.

"Iaquinta," he'd say, "I am not going to spoon-feed you through residency."

The next morning he canceled a scheduled cancer operation. We already had the patient on the table and had begun removing her thyroid cancer when Dr. Organ discovered the gynecologists were going to remove the metastatic disease after we finished. But, Dr. Organ refused to let them operate.

"It's not going to happen; I wasn't informed of this decision. When was this decided?" Dr. Organ stood erect, looking down at the much shorter Corey over the patient's open neck.

"Two days ago, sir," Corey answered quietly.

"Nobody told me about this. The second half's canceled."

I didn't understand. Dr. Organ wasn't required to be in the room for the second half. What difference did it make to him? How did this interfere with his day? He had no other cases to follow. If the plan didn't benefit the patient he should have explained why.

Corey didn't understand either. He pleaded his case, but Dr. Organ insisted there was none.

Corey and I closed in silent frustration. Hey, we're the future of American medicine, remember? Now's your chance, teach us something. But nothing happened. Dr. Organ stripped off his gown and strode out of the room in his usual fashion.

Dr. Organ exemplified the difference between admiration and respect. He was admirable, just as a professional athlete is. It is admirable to catch more touchdown passes than anyone else. Children aspire to replicate these feats.

But this in no way implies respect. That same athlete could be arrested for using crack cocaine or found guilty of rape. Not at all respectable.

134

It is admirable that some surgeons have devoted their lives to the practice of medicine. But this does not mean they are respectable people. They can live comfortably in ignorance, because nobody will ever tell them the difference. Dr. Organ can be King of the Hospital for the rest of his life, but it will be Corey that I respect for throwing that extra stitch into the dude with the perforated ulcer. That patient did great after his operation.

At least this patient would get radioactive iodine to treat her metastatic disease.

Chapter 25

Rachel called to tell me that she was going to apply to do her Masters in public health at UC Berkeley. She needed to take an extra year during or after medical school to get her Masters so that she could go into epidemiology and infectious disease.

"Don't come out here just for me," I replied. I didn't even have to wait for the pause in conversation to know I just destroyed what could have been a great moment. I couldn't help it. It was a reflexive response. But I didn't stop.

"I knew this girl who chose a college just because it was where her boyfriend went. A couple of months into the year they broke up and she didn't know what she was doing there."

It struck me that Rachel expected me to be at least somewhat excited when she said, "I thought you'd be at least somewhat excited."

Oops.

I am a moron. I assumed she hadn't already thought about everything I had just said. She was a big girl; she knew how to make her own decision.

"I don't see how our relationship could develop if we don't spend more time together," she said, "and I need to get my Masters."

"You're right. It'd be pathetic if we broke up just because of distance. It will be better if you come and find out what's wrong with me."

She didn't say, "I'm getting the idea." But she should have.

I didn't want her to not to come. I didn't want her coming just to be with me. But, if we didn't, there would be that "what if" scenario to play over and over in my head over the next few years. There is nothing worse than a "what if" scenario.

I consulted one of my married friends. I hesitated to call him. A doctor calling an organic chemist for relationship advice? Sounds like the beginning of a bad joke. But he was a married man; he had to have something to offer. His first response was, "Way to go, Mr. Fear of Commitment."

"I'm not afraid of committing," I said. "I'm afraid of committing to the wrong person. I wouldn't be able to deal with thinking I made a mistake two years after the fact." I didn't want to waste her time. I didn't want the guilt of having her put so much effort into us being

136

together.

During medical school, a couple of my friends got married. I asked them, separately, how they knew they were marrying the right person. They just looked at me like I was an idiot and replied, "You just know."

That's the feeling I wanted, and I wasn't there yet.

Chapter 26

Day 91. Yes! The 25% mark. One fourth of the way through the year. The clock does not stop.

I celebrated the occasion by staying on call over the weekend. I spent a considerable time with one patient, Mrs. Hughes. She always greeted me with a smile and, despite being forty, possessed the serenity of a great grandmother. Her gleaming white teeth stood out against her dark skin and stood out because a perfect set of ivories were rare in County Hospital. Her daughters often flanked her side, bearing the same smile.

We admitted her for a possible bowel obstruction or appendicitis. She hadn't been having bowel movements and had a physical exam consistent with appendicitis; however, she didn't have a fever or elevated white blood count. Her CT scan two weeks earlier had looked normal. The morning after admission a barium enema didn't show any obvious abnormalities. Why weren't things moving, through?

Dr. Organ stayed home on Saturdays, so we couldn't wave her past his eyes and have him spit out the diagnosis. So she remained an "interesting case." The last thing a patient wants to be is an interesting case. If the doctor feels obligated to share your situation with others, be wary. Interesting cases often turn out to be rare tumors, freakish anomalies, or just plain inexplicable.

On Sunday, she seemed better. She had a normal bowel movement thanks to the cathartic properties of barium. We decided to let her drink liquids.

A few hours later, I stopped by her room. She winced and pointed at her bloated abdomen. I, of course, prodded it. I thought I could feel a small mass in her right lower quadrant of her abdomen. It could be an enlarged appendix.

I offered to put down an NG tube. A nasogastric tube is literally up your nose with a rubber hose. The hose suctions out the stomach contents to reduce pain and bloating. She agreed, cheerful and eager to undergo whatever torture I had in mind to help cure her. There are a number of ways to hurt people in an attempt to make them better; for example, just to deliver anesthesia I stick them with a needle.

The secret to passing an NG tube is to remember that the nasal passage goes straight back, even slightly downward, from the nostril. If you shove the tube up you won't get anything but a bloody nose and a sore patient.

When I approached her holding the plastic tube in my hand she said, "I'm not so sure I should have agreed to this."

I hesitated.

"No, go ahead. It needs to be done," she assured me.

She wriggled as I inserted the tube into her nose. She gagged as I advanced it. I let up on the pressure.

"Swallow," I commanded.

She swallowed weakly and I attempted to advance the tube. The tube irritated her airway and she went into a coughing fit.

I pulled the tube back and then all the way out as she hacked. A giant wad of phlegm shot past me, missing me by inches. By ninety-one days I knew to never align myself within firing range of any bodily orifice.

I hated torturing people. I went to find some anesthetic spray to numb her throat. It might seem cruel that I didn't administer the numbing spray preemptively, but usually the tube passes easily. I sprayed the back of her throat and gave it a few seconds to work. She nodded for me to give it another try. But the tube wouldn't pass.

This only happens to two types of people: the really nice ones and the absolute creeps.

"Try drinking this water through a straw," I said. "As you are swallowing, I will pass the tube." Maybe she was focusing on it too much.

"Anything it takes to get this done," she said. I loved her attitude. Maybe she had it all in perspective already. She did have kids after all, vaginal delivery—there wasn't a C-section scar on her abdomen.

I put the tube into her left nostril and felt it slide in with little resistance. I had her start swallowing and I felt the tube hit the back of her pharynx and turn downward. Then it slid easily down the esophagus, getting pulled with every swallow. When it reached the stomach I flipped the suction on. The tube immediately filled with dark green liquid. A liter of bile-stained fluid filled the clear plastic container. Her body relaxed with relief.

I excused myself to page Corey. "Mrs. Hughes is obstructed. I think we should explore her." He agreed, but said Dr. Fagan wanted to get a colonoscopy on Monday instead. (Dr. Fagan enjoyed calls from home even though he was covering for Dr. Organ.) But Corey had me do the right thing. I pre-opped her just in case.

"Hey man, while you're at it can you get radiology to do a needle-guided biopsy of the guy with the abdominal mass?" Corey asked.

"Sure." He might as well have asked me to part the Red Sea. I ordered a series of abdominal x-rays on Mrs. Hughes just to confirm my suspicions. Then, I headed down to the radiology department.

I learned quickly to bring the requests directly to the radiologist myself. The written requests were always denied or "never received," much like lab requests. The hospital's gremlins work tirelessly to ensure things "get lost."

The radiologists needed to be approached delicately. I couldn't figure out if they were generally lazy or tremendously overworked. Either way, they never acquiesced to any procedure request without a battle.

I entered their lair. Light boxes filled three walls of the rooms. One radiologist sat with his back to me, looking at his wall of films.

"Good afternoon," I offered.

He glanced at me and went back to his films. I didn't fool him. He knew I didn't stop by just to say good afternoon.

"I have a patient that needs a CT-guided needle biopsy."

"No." Reflex response. The films were still in my hand. He hadn't even looked at them. He clicked on his Dictaphone on and started reading the x-ray in front of him.

I have no desire to grease elbows and wax egos otherwise I would have gone into used car sales. I only wanted one thing: to get this job done.

Wait. Rewind. Time for the Jedi Mind Trick.

"This patient is not an operative candidate, and I don't even know if you could biopsy this mass. It's really in there." I hoped his ego would take the bait.

The radiologist turned and snatched the films from me. He threw them up on the wall on his left. "Oh yeah, I can hit this, no problem. I'll do it tomorrow, about 9."

"Thanks."

And that, folks, is the Art of Medicine.

140

Then, I checked Mrs. Hughes' films. The air-fluid levels proved she was obstructed. I pre-opped her, but she looked much better than before I had put the tube down. Of course, she had two fewer liters of green fluid festering in her gut.

I explained to her that we would open her abdomen and find the point of obstruction. I told her it might require us to remove a segment of bowel to relieve it. In a worst-case scenario she might even need a colostomy bag. I told her I hoped that inflammation caused the problem, but it could be cancer.

Practicing medicine supported my pessimistic attitude. You want your doctor to think the worst of you. You don't want the optimist doc who thinks it would be a weird presentation for a heart attack . . . Naw, it couldn't be. He looks so healthy I won't even check the labs.

No, you want a pessimist. I better make sure that lump isn't cancer; so what if she's not a smoker. There aren't many rules, but the first is to make sure the patient is going to die before you figure out what's wrong. If I could rule out the killers, I had time to figure the rest out. Last thing I want is your relatives to sue me just because you didn't leave a large enough inheritance.

I told her the plan. We needed to "run her bowel," which meant feed it between a finger and thumb, looking/feeling for a mass. Of course, I didn't say it that way to her. No. We needed to "explore" her to "evaluate the cause of obstruction." Lady, the truth is we are going to slice you from stem to stern Freddy-Krueger style. Then we're going to muck around your intestines looking for the culprit. But I refrained from scaring the bejesus out of her.

When I was all done explaining, I asked if she had any questions.

"No. I trust you. I put my life in your hands."

"We'll do the best we can for you," I replied. "I'll see you in a little while." I turned out into the hallway. My life in your hands. She had just met me yesterday. Who was I that she could comfortably say this to? How could the letters "MD" mean that much? What a scary idea.

Maybe that's what MD was supposed to mean. Practicing medicine meant knowing how to care for people stuck in situations where they couldn't care for themselves. Doctors were supposed to be trusted to take lives into their hands.

Such high stakes. Human lives. No room for the inevitable errors. And she placed all this responsibility on someone who owned a collection of unopened Star Wars figures. Med schools need to be far more rigorous with the application process.

In the first year of medical school, one of the professors told us that we would all kill at least one person. We would miss a diagnosis; treat the wrong thing. It was a sobering thought. An unfair thought. I was expected to be 100% my entire career in a society where people cheered if their favorite baseball player hit .333.

When we opened her abdomen, a busy hive of cancer greeted us. The queen mother was on the right colon. Tiny babies, too small for any scan, decorated the small intestine, uterus, ovaries, and omentum. Lesions infiltrated her liver. Her prognosis went from bad to miserable. Six months...maybe.

I wanted to vomit. A forty-year-old woman had come into the OR with a stomachache and was going to leave with a death sentence. She put her life in my hands and I couldn't do anything with it.

*

When I got home that night I called my mom, probably just to make sure she didn't have a stomachache.

"Oh, I've had a hectic day," she said. "I had two cases this morning. Then, I met Lisa for lunch. We chatted too long and I had to rush back to the office to meet clients. I didn't get out of there until 5:30. I sped over to the gym to do my workout. Then, I came home and was too tired to watch the movie I rented, so I've just been resting."

I wanted to scream, "You call that a BAD day?" I wanted that day. I didn't want to be telling a young woman she had incurable cancer. I wanted to work out, have a long lunch with a friend, and the opportunity to lounge. I resisted my temptation to invalidate her feelings by telling her about my last 48 hours.

"Well, hopefully tomorrow will be better for you," I said. If she said she had a hectic day, then she had a hectic day.

After our conversation, I had an epiphany. Surgeons' marriages failed precisely due to that lack of perspective. After a grueling day at the hospital with delayed cases, rude patients, being humiliated by staff doctors and nurses, and add-on cases, the surgeon had to go home and be the same compassionate man his wife married. When his wife said she had a terrible day with their three-year-old son, it meant she did. She wanted sympathy. To disregard it and say how much worse his day was would belittle her. It would mean that her day, and her feelings, didn't count. A marriage couldn't last long if this episode repeated itself often.

That was the trick. Don't try to make others understand. Leave everything behind at the hospital. It will be waiting for you the next morning, and if it can't wait, they'll page you.

Chapter 27

INTERMISSION: FREE MEDICAL ADVICE

Share this information with anyone you know.

Don't clean your car naked, especially if your vibrator is on the seat. It might get stuck up your butt.

A thin sock is not a form of birth control.

Don't store your shampoo in a syrup bottle. You might slip in the shower and lodge Aunt Jemima halfway up your butt.

Do not insert devices that blow compressed air into your rectum.

Mountain Dew does not really make boys sterile.

Do not allow devices that suck air to be put into your rectum.

Don't sit on light bulbs naked. They might "slip in."

Putting breast milk into your baby's ear won't cure his ear infection.

Do not stick your penis in a three-liter bottle just to see if it fits.

Do not inhale Legos.

Do not let your partner fill your vagina with strawberries.

If you must have your vagina filled with strawberries count how many go in, and, of course, count how many are taken out.

Saran Wrap is not a form of birth control (for either boys or girls).

Coca-Cola is not a form of birth control, even if it is flushed into the vagina.

Don't touch sharp metal parts just to see if they are sharp. Or hot objects just to see if they are hot.

Do not clean lawn equipment naked.

If a tooth falls out, don't jam it into your ear canal for safekeeping.

Do not ignore that festering thing growing on your skin for the last five years.

Do not jam chunks of crayons into your ears.

Never clean your ears with a Q-tip while driving down a bumpy road.

Do not plug your ears with gum to keep the bugs out.

And, no, it doesn't take seven years to digest gum. Not even seven days.

Your "healer" might have good intentions, but gargling your urine every morning might not be the best way to cure your sore throat.

Do not try to lance your own hemorrhoids.

Do not swallow hundreds of carpet tacks.

Do not swallow whole pork chop bones.

Do not swallow staple removers. Yes, the big clampy remover.

A uterus is supposed to be an internal organ. If it is hanging out do not just push it back in. Go see your local physician.

The rectum is supposed to be an internal organ. If it is hanging out do not just push it back in and do your plowing while standing up on the tractor for two days. Instead, go see your local physician.

Chances are a testicle the size of an orange will not go back to normal on its own. Go to a doctor.

Do not stick the arm of your glasses into your urethra. It might break off, lodging itself within your penis.

If you find little magnets on the ground on your way home, don't shove them into your nostrils.

Do not leave a rubber band on your penis for two days.

Do not use a metal pipe as an erectile aid.

Do not light your cigarette with your supplemental oxygen blowing in your face. In fact, if you require an oxygen tank to breathe, you shouldn't smoke.

Do not insist that the only thing you ate was a handful of little peppermint candies when they were indeed hundreds of pebbles.

After you finish eating popcorn, do not pick your teeth with a stick pin (with the ball on the end) and accidentally inhale it.

Chop a hot dog into tiny pieces before feeding it to a two year old.

Do not pee on electric fences.

Although the people in health food stores are knowledgeable, it is unlikely they can cure your cancer with herbal remedies.

When your car stops dead on a dark night, do not check to see if there is gas in the tank by lighting a match and removing the gas cap.

Don't tell your girlfriend not to come out to California just because you are there.

Chapter 28

Rachel visited for the weekend.

I stopped to get her flowers before picking her up at the airport. Then I parked my car and went in to meet her. That's true love. I spied her coming down the hallway and hid behind a kiosk. When she passed I snuck up behind her. It's funny to look at people who are expecting to see you any minute. She looked determined. Maybe she was thinking about getting her luggage.

She got onto the moving walkway. I crept up right behind her and started to infringe on her personal space, just over her left shoulder. She moved away slightly without looking. I inched closer. She gave one of those narrow-eyed glances women give freaky men. Then she did a double take.

"Creep," she exclaimed. Now she was smiling. "How long have you been following me?"

I had achieved a personal victory. It's hard to get someone to fly cross-country and then call you a creep the first moment they see you. Try it sometime.

The flowers made everything okay.

We had a great weekend. We watched her favorite childhood movie, "Watership Down." We went to the art museum. We didn't talk about my failure on the phone. We played kickball. Okay, we didn't really play kickball; we didn't have enough people. But we kicked around my kickball. Then we made cookies. I have a great recipe for lemon macadamia nut white chocolate chip cookies.

I don't know when she noticed, but Rachel finally said something.

"Will you stop it?"

"Stop what?"

"Stop scraping that bowl."

"If I get this last bit out I can probably double the size of that last cookie." I almost had the bowl cleaner than before we started.

"You're neurotic. The scraping is driving me nuts. You've got enough."

I couldn't stand wasting food. When I ate yogurt I scraped the container clean. When I added a stick of butter to the cookie batter I scraped the wrapper clean. Those things counted. The manufacturer put one cup of butter in that wrapper. The recipe called for one cup; I needed what was left on that wrapper.

Besides, people were starving in Africa. If I didn't clean my plate, then over the year I'd be throwing away what could have fed a family of five.

I guess that proved that I needed Rachel. I needed someone who could put up with my neuroses. I needed someone to prevent me from becoming a full-blown psychotic.

I knew I couldn't predict the future and that worried me. But by the end of her visit I knew that I enjoyed the present with her. True, we might despise each other in six months. But why care? That allotted me six months of good times.

I needed to push my pessimism aside to tell her how I felt. But I didn't.

Chapter 29

I would have rather been kicked in the groin than be stuck in the hospital that morning. Heading back to work after a weekend with Rachel still packed the same punch it did the first time around. I wondered if Corey felt that way every morning on his way to work after spending the previous evening with his family. Too bad Dr. Organ was standing across the OR table, or I would have asked.

As it was, Dr. Organ seemed content on badgering Corey about bowel cancer, which left me to daydream. I needed the ability to teleport. I could live anywhere and go anywhere. Ideally, I could transport my clothes and anything else I held, including other people. How cool would it be to zap over to the Taj Mahal for the afternoon? I could zap myself to Madison to have dinner with Rachel. That would obviate her needing to take a year off of med school. I should have been a wizard instead of a surgeon.

Dr. Organ eased up on verbally abusing Corey and started operating. He didn't say much, but watching him operate was a lesson in itself. He didn't waste a single motion, which is the ultimate goal of every surgeon. The operation should be as efficient as it is effective. Dr. Organ made surgery look like tying your shoes.

I watched the two of them "unzip" the abdomen of an 88-year-old woman with a bowel obstruction. As soon as he could get hits mitts in, Corey started running the bowel.

"What's this? It feels like...rocks." Corey held up a segment of dilated bowel and I felt little beads between my fingers. Corey milked some back into the stomach.

The anesthetist flipped the NG tube on suction. Little pebbles flew up the tube and rattled around the suction canister before clogging it. What were pebbles doing in her intestines?

"Maybe she has pica," I offered. Pica is an appetite perversion, like a child eating dirt. It can be seen in people with iron deficiency or mental disturbances.

When Rachel was little, she had been tested for pica. She ate anything and everything. She gnawed a hole in the backseat of her dad's car. She ate paint. She was the Castor Oil poster child.

I liked that she was a weirdo too.

Corey milked the rest of the pebbles out of the small intestine and into the large colon. This would allow them to pass in her stool. She

148

didn't require any further operation. Dr. Organ didn't have any witty comments. He just shook his head, perplexed. "All right guys, close up."

I wanted to call out after him, "Common things are common."

When the patient awoke she vehemently denied eating pebbles. She said, "The only thing I ate was peppermint candies. You know, they have those little stones in them."

What little stones? The specks of flavor? Maybe she ate those peppermint-flavored pebbles.

Regardless, she pooped pebbles. Pebble Pooper.

PART 2: THE PRIVATE HOSPITAL

Chapter 30

I figured out their modus operandi. As soon as I got used to something, they changed everything. After three months I understood the county system, so they threw me into a private hospital with new paperwork, new rules, and a new chief. I was paired with John, Corey's good friend and co-chief.

The month started on a Friday, which gave the two of us one day to learn the place before being left alone on Saturday to man the ship. The next morning I floundered my way through rounds, barely able to navigate the byzantine structure. No one builds a hospital for the future; they are built to operate at maximum capacity the day they open. Then, additions are added as afterthoughts connected by tunnels and bridges so that the map of the place looks like a flowchart on steroids. Clearly, a boy with an ant farm fetish designed the hospital.

But I soon learned that I'd survive, and maybe even enjoy, working in Walnut Creek Hospital.

"Doctor, do you need some help?" A pert nurse appeared to be talking to me. She must have mistaken me for a human.

"What?" I glanced over my shoulder to look for a real doctor.

"What are you looking for? Maybe I could get it for you."

What the hell is going on here? You want to help me? You're joking, right? I told her I was looking for some dressing supplies.

She looked at me like I had just insulted her. She had already changed his dressing this morning.

"You already did it?" I had to hear it twice to believe it.

"Yes, the orders are for twice a day."

I think I felt what my dad felt the first time he saw me shovel the snow from the front walk. Wait, he can do that? And do it well? Then I don't have to do it—not today, and maybe not ever again.

The hospital's pleasant atmosphere helped offset our hard work. The grueling call days happened just as often and with more cases than County.

We started Saturday morning by being dumped a "chole" (slang for cholecystectomy, which is the removal of the gallbladder) and a pacemaker implantation left over from the night before. Last night's surgeon had worked straight through the night with too many cases to finish. John went to insert the pacemaker and sent me to see the gallbladder. But before I had a chance to see him the ER doc called me to "rule out" appendicitis.

It's amazing how quickly things had become rote. Do racecar drivers think it's just another race? A few months ago I would have been excited, but now it was just appendicitis.

The patient looked my age. That freaked me out, because I couldn't envision him as my doctor. No way he'd cut out *my* appendix. No, he looked like the slightly disheveled guy getting over his obsession with grunge rock. He still watched *The Simpsons* and anxiously awaited the release of the next Playstation.

If he thought the same, he didn't tell me. That tipped me off that he belonged in the ER. The "social" visitors are the ones who complained about my age.

The guy looked relaxed enough. The problem with having the head of the bed up is that it makes everyone look like they are lounging. I have a hard time taking loungers seriously.

He told me his stomachache woke him up in the middle of the night. Then he felt crampy, nauseated, and ran to the bathroom and puked.

That got my attention. Not the puke, the part about pain waking him up from sleep. Suspicious.

"What'd you have for dinner?"

"Fish. Caught it, cleaned it, and cooked it myself." He smiled the smile of a proud fisherman.

Had he given himself food poisoning? Or was his fish story a red herring? I dismissed the fish as a decoy and decided to make Dr. Organ proud by obtaining more history. "Anything else unusual yesterday?"

"No, but the evening before last I went swimming in a contaminated reservoir. I didn't see the 'No Swimming: Animal Waste Contamination' sign until afterward."

He reminded me of a medical school test patient. He had a school of herring. Did he have an infection causing gastroenteritis? Next, he'd tell me he just returned from rural Africa and might have inhaled a parasite.

I welcomed the opportunity to be the Sherlock Holmes of

151

Bowelsville. Time to solve a mystery. I set about examining the scene of the crime.

The suspect rested comfortably, apparently not in too much pain. His messed-up hair meant it hurt enough to skip grooming before coming in. He obviously didn't live with my mom. When I broke my arm, she made me take a bath before going to the hospital.

He had a mild elevation of temperature, but not a true fever. A fever is 101.5; he was a mere 99.8. Curious, but non-specific. I had him lay down on the exam table. We call it an exam table because to call that lightly padded rock a "bed" would open us up to malpractice.

I tapped on his abdomen. He complained everywhere hurt, but when I pushed on his right lower quadrant he squirmed. Aha! He was most tender right at his appendix. Very suspicious.

I checked his labs. His white blood cell count was slightly elevated. Hmm, possibly an early presentation of appendicitis. I expected him to be in more pain. Someone with true peritoneal irritation will lie absolutely still.

Time to report my suspect to John: early appendicitis.

He saw the patient and repeated everything I did, much to the chagrin of the patient.

"It's our nature not to trust each other," I shrugged.

John excused us from the room. He thought it was gastroenteritis.

I countered with early appendicitis.

"Sure, but this guy could go home and come back in twelve hours with an exam more indicative of appendicitis, or he could be fine."

"You're right. But why would I want to operate on him at midnight instead of noon?" I still liked my sleep, even if I rarely saw any.

John grinned. "Now you're thinking, Sally-boy, but it doesn't do us any good if he has gastroenteritis. You go set up that gallbladder. I'll call the ol' attending and see what he thinks."

I rushed upstairs. Getting the man with gallstones ready for surgery didn't involve any sleuthing. But maybe I'd get to do the case—a laparoscopic cholecystectomy. I could pretend that I was a tiny man in the abdomen and the cautery tool was my flamethrower. It was my job to dissect the parasitic gallbladder off the host liver.

My pager went off—an unfamiliar number, which meant another

consult. A medicine doctor had a patient with gallstone pancreatitis that had improved and was now ready to have her gallbladder removed. That made two gallbladders. A perfect set-up for the surgery adage of "see one, do one, teach one."

By the time I got to the second gallbladder, I had the routine down. I'm sure I set a land speed record. "Hi, I'm-doctor-Iaquinta-from-the-surgery-service-your-doctor-tells-me-you-are-getting-over-your-pancreatitis-and-has-asked-me-to-evaluate-you-for-surgical-removal-of-your-gallbladder-I'm-just-going-to-examine-you-while-I-ask-you-a-few-questions."

When I finished consenting him, I took a breath. But just when I finished my pager went off like clockwork. Another ICU patient needed a pacemaker placed. Everything was happening in twos as if we were loading up the Ark with two of every kind of sickness.

Then, the attending paged. He thought the guy in the ER should go to the OR for an appy. He also wanted to meet the two men with gallstones. So, as a team, we went to see them. It's usually women who get cholelithiasis, better known as gallstones. There is a mnemonic called the five Fs. The stereotypical gallstone patient is female, fat, forty, fertile, and flatulent.

On the way John asked me, "Do you think that guy has appendicitis?"

"Yep. The end of his appendix will be sticking up like a sore thumb."

"No way. It's going to be a normal appendix. Want to bet on it?"

"Sure."

"What do you want to bet?" The added excitement of a bet made John grin widely.

"Let's just bet."

"We have to bet something. How about a buck?"

"A buck?" Why just a buck?

"Okay, a quarter."

"Fine." We shook on it. Did he think a dollar was out of my league?

John proved the denomination didn't matter. "You just lost 25 cents. Sucker." He danced around behind the attending. For a second I knew what it was like to have an older brother.

Dr. Bergman smiled. He supported my bet by taking the patient to the OR. We stopped by to see the two guys with gallstones. Both had the TV tuned into "The Price is Right." That was another difference from County Hospital. Over there everyone watched "Jerry Springer," if the TV worked.

On our way to the OR our attending told us, "There's a woman in 242 I want you guys to take a look at. It might be a consult out of desperation. I'll leave it to the two of you."

Attendings don't leave the residents the exciting cases.

He ditched us, leaving John and me unhindered. We perused 242's chart. It's always best to fill yourself with as much misleading information as possible before seeing the patient. She had been admitted two days before for abdominal pain. Unimpressive labs. Equally unimpressive vital signs. Any films?

Someone noted she couldn't get a CT scan because she exceeded the scanner's weight limit.

John looked at me, eyes bulging, "I think the weight limit is 400 pounds!"

"Whoa."

"The weird thing is when you see a CT of these huge people you realize they are actually normal people trapped inside a giant layer of fat. All their organs and their abdominal cavity are the same size as skinny people. It's strange."

The lady filled the whole hospital bed. I thought of her as a skinny woman carrying two of me draped over her shoulders. I could have been carved off of her, like a butcher taking off a slab of bacon.

Her rotund husband squashed the chair next to her. Together they weighed a family of five.

John and I silently sighed with relief as we heard her story. We wouldn't have to experience the nightmare of operating on her. The opening incision needs to be huge in order to get enough exposure into the abdomen. In addition, obese people have poor oxygen reserves, which can make them susceptible to complications. Their normal-sized lungs work extra hard to supply oxygen to their massive bodies. Then, because of the skin creases, the poor hygiene that goes with creases, and the poor blood flow, they get wound infections.

John asked the big question. "How much do you weigh?"

"410 pounds." Just over the scanner's limit. If we kept her NPO (nil per os, or, nothing by mouth) she'd lose that weight in short time.

"I think your biggest problem right now is your weight. It prevents us from fully evaluating you," John informed her. "I don't think you have a surgical problem, but the CT scan would have been helpful to determine that earlier. As for your weight, it will continue to be a problem even if your abdominal pain resolves. I see that you have a history of emphysema. You are stressing your lungs to try to keep up with your oxygen demand."

"I know I need to lose weight. I want to get my stomach banded so I get full quicker," she said quietly.

I shrunk back into the corner of the room. John continued a lecture that seemed to be a weird parallel to Corey's drug-shooting lecture back at County Hospital. But instead of drugs, the suburbanites die of fat.

At just the moment the steam started coming out of her husband's ears, John wrapped up his talk. We raced out of her room on to the next victim.

John picked up on my discomfort. "You are not wrong to tell a patient what they need to know. I can't ignore her obesity when it is the root of her problems." He paused for a second. "And don't back down just because it makes her husband mad. It's your job to tell the patient what's wrong, even if no one wants to hear it."

I understood his point. Obesity is a disease. It has nothing to do with aesthetics. Overeating is a bad habit, an addiction. We tell smokers to quit smoking. Fat people should quit eating.

By the way, obese is a medical term. Sometimes patients see their chart and are offended that they are referred to as obese. This has even been used against doctors in lawsuits in showing just how "uncaring they are." Obese is defined as a body mass index greater than 30. Body mass index is weight (in kilograms) divided by height (in meters) squared.

Just then I was interrupted by another page. Another consult: possible perirectal abscess. My favorite.

"Ohhh, butt pus, butt pus, butt pus," John chanted. He has a thing about butt pus. Just the mention of it triggers that chant. "I can't wait until next year. I'll never have to deal with butt pus again." John had received a Plastic and Reconstructive Surgery fellowship.

"Nor will I." I headed toward the ER and John left me for the OR.

One of the real reasons I wanted to go into ENT over other types of surgery is that I hate doing vaginal and rectal exams. Believe me, there is absolutely nothing exciting about having to do these exams. I imagine some guys might think it would be cool to see naked women and vice versa. First of all, the hospital setting, the gown, and the sickness remove any attractive qualities. Second, the reason for the exam is to rule out disease. This implies you often rule in disease. Let it be known sailors' jokes underestimate the malodorous stench of some genital infections.

The rectal exam, also a subject of many jokes, could not be a source of excitement. The first things discovered upon spreading someone's cheeks are their wiping hygiene and if they have external hemorrhoids. Neither of these are things I care to know about anyone. Then I have to put my finger in their brownstar and feel around. Sometimes poop comes out on my fingertip. Then I smear it on a card to see if there is blood in it. I've always wanted to exclaim, mid-exam, to a patient, "Oh my God! My hand's stuck," as I do the rectal, but I fear it would end my medical career.

This sort of thing isn't in the medical school brochure. My pay averages out to about five dollars an hour. I deserved a much higher rate to stick my finger up someone's butt. Hookers charge more.

I performed the exam. No signs of infection. No pus, redness, swelling, or tenderness. Another dandy anus. I couldn't figure out why they had called me. Those buttheads.

The problem with seeing consults in the ER is that the ER physicians see you. Invariably, someone else wants to "bounce something off you." Didn't they know the more they bounced off of me, the later they delayed my lunch?

"So you didn't think that guy had an abscess?" a short ER doctor with a gray toupee asked.

"No. I didn't find anything on exam."

"Well, I've got this woman with a possible incarcerated hernia. I've been trying to reduce it for fifteen minutes. Maybe you could come take a look at it?"

Didn't he know to wait until I was down to the cafeteria before consulting me? He must not have known I was an intern.

An incarcerated hernia is a true surgical emergency. If a section of

156

bowel or other visceral contents herniates through the abdominal wall and can't be reduced, it can cut off its own blood supply. Because the bowel is loaded with bacteria, dead bowel quickly becomes infected bowel.

She was a pleasant woman. Gray hair, glasses, 62, and a husband at her side. "I had this painful lump in my side. I still feel it, but it doesn't hurt anymore. My doctor, Dr. Childs—do you know Dr. Childs? What a nice doctor. Dr. Childs told me I have a hernia that I need to get fixed."

"Why didn't you?"

"Oh, me and Bob went to visit our kids in Oregon for the last two weeks. I figured I'd get it done as soon as we have things straightened out around the house."

People's priorities boggle me. In the county hospital people couldn't get early healthcare, but the middle class gets to prioritize their lives and come in whenever it's convenient. Either way, the emergency rooms stay full.

I shoved on the firm knot of tissue just below her umbilicus, and she let out a loud yelp. Once again the white coat proved it was permission to torture strangers.

I told her I'd put an ice pack on it and be back in fifteen minutes. I learned that trick from John. Most of what I learned had trickled down from the other residents. Nobody puts the cool stuff in books.

Time to get some food. We didn't have a meal plan at this hospital, but we got to raid the cafeteria for extra patient food. I couldn't imagine anything worse than the patient meals, which made it perfect for a starving intern with no other options. The visitor cafeteria offered food of equally low quality, but you had to pay a king's ransom for it. This wasn't one of the hospitals that had been invaded by a franchise restaurant. Hospitals are the one place where fast food restaurants should be—this way they can rush you from the dining room to the cardiac catheterization lab when you have your heart attack.

As I left the patient's room, one of the ER doctors pulled me aside. "I just saw a man that I think you need to evaluate." He paused.

If he thought I was going to bite on that alone, I wanted to know what he was smoking. Didn't he know his partner in crime had already tagged me twice this hour? I raised an eyebrow and gave him a nod of encouragement.

That got him back on track. "This is a forty-two year old man with a history of a perirectal abscess. It was surgically drained four weeks and six weeks ago. He comes back complaining of persistent pain and discharge. I don't feel anything on exam, but I thought you should check it out just to make sure." Then he tacked on, "He does have pus coming from his rectum."

Okay, two things wrong with that. The first is, you said, "Check it out just to make sure." I am not the come-check-it-out-just-to-make-sure consultant. I want to operate. Call me for the people that need to be cut open. If you don't think it's anything, send the patient home. The second problem is butt pus. Did everything have to happen in twos today?

"It's a good sign that it is draining; makes it less likely we need to cut anything open." I liked to give the ER doctors a little preliminary opinion of the situation. A subtle way of preparing them for the future, as in I'm probably going to leave him and his nasty ass in your care. And before he had time to get defensive, I added, "Thanks, I'll go see him right away."

The man had a recurrent perirectal infection. When I spread his cheeks apart there was yellowish-green pus draining from his anus. It was one of those sights that would stick with me the rest of my life, like seeing the Great Pyramids...only juicier.

I could feel a lump in his rectum, but it felt like it had a groove in it. I wasn't sure. I continued to probe until I realized my fingers just weren't long enough. And my hand was just too big. I followed my digital exam with an anoscopic exam, which entails putting a clear plastic tube past the anal sphincter to get a look inside. It's like snorkeling, only less fish. I saw some pus and a little ulceration, but nothing else.

I told him I'd have one of the other surgeons take a look.

But he had his own plans. "I only came here to get antibiotics. I don't want surgery. I've had this before and there's no way I am going through surgery again." It wasn't a statement; it was threat. He was a big guy, too.

Him saying that pretty much guaranteed he would require surgery. That's the way people jinx themselves. This was going to be fun.

I paged John. "Is it BUTT PUS?"

"How about 'hello?'"

"Come on, is it BUTT PUS?"

158

"Yup, lots of it, just for you."

"Really?

"Yeah, it's already draining. But you can still put your finger in it." He said he'd be right down. It was hard to hear his enthusiasm over the sounds of the football game he was watching.

As I waited, one of the ER docs, the short one with the mustache and dopey voice, pulled me aside once again. "I have a patient that I think has a bowel obstruction. He has air fluid levels on x-ray and hyperactive bowel sounds. He has been having diarrhea."

Wait a minute. Maybe we don't speak the same language. "If he's been having diarrhea it doesn't sound like an obstruction."

"But…"

The ER doc was eager to protest, but I didn't let him start. "What room is he in?"

I had a feeling this was going to be another bogus consult, either out of laziness or ignorance. It was probably the only thing he could think of to keep me from going to the cafeteria. I grabbed the patient's chart out of the rack and headed toward his room. I saw his films outside the door. There weren't any air-fluid levels. I checked the name on the chart and the x-rays twice. No mistake. The chart said, "77-year-old male with diffuse abdominal pain, diarrhea, nausea, and vomiting since last night." I knew exactly what the diagnosis was…a lazy ER doc.

The man had one of those nasally voices. It sounded like he had been a lifelong helium abuser. He looked dehydrated, but then it might have just been all his wrinkly skin. He told me his pain had been improving during the day. He had thrown up once the night before and had about twelve episodes of diarrhea during the day. It was profuse and watery.

It sounded like gastroenteritis. His benign exam included me doing yet another rectal exam on a normal butt. Had the ER doc even seen him before consulting me? I couldn't find his note.

John had better get down here quickly, I thought, so we can get out of the ER doctors' sight.

Not a minute later, he came strolling into the ER. With a disappointed smirk he reached into his pocket and handed me a quarter.

"Yes." I clenched the quarter in my fist and held it above my head like an Olympic champion.

"Oh, it was hardly inflamed. I'm just giving this to you." Of course John would never admit true defeat.

He saw the butt pus man and thought a course of antibiotics would be an acceptable alternative to more surgery. The patient latched onto the plan wholeheartedly as neither party seemed keen on draining butt pus that evening.

Then, John agreed the other man had gastroenteritis. Chalk up another one for Sherlock. And by the time our attending came down to see the woman with the hernia, it had slid back into place; so, there was no need for emergency surgery.

Dr. Bergman managed to slip out of the ER, but John and I were roped back in by one of the internal medicine docs seeing a consult. "I just saw this woman who I think has a surgical abdomen. I was called to see her regarding a possible urosepsis, but that's not her problem. Her urine isn't that dirty. But her lower abdomen is diffusely tender. She said she had a little bit of diarrhea but hasn't been moving her bowels well. Her plain film shows a lot of gas."

John looked past her at the x-rays. "Did you do a rectal?"

"Yes, it was normal. Guaiac negative." No blood. Cancer can cause occult blood.

I looked at the film. Gas inflated the loops of bowel. But none of it reached the rectum.

"See this?" John asked, waving his hand over the pelvis. "There is something here. It's too opaque."

I hadn't seen it until he pointed it out. The lower pelvis did have a diffuse opacity greater than normal. That something was likely causing the blockage. In old people it often ends up being impacted stool. It's cured by digitally (meaning with a finger, not electronically) disimpacting the clogged pipe. Not something on my bucket list.

Another 77-year-old. We really were loading the Ark.

The woman was one big wrinkle. Her deep wrinkles made me imagine her once being twice as large.

She didn't say hello. She didn't look at us. She didn't want to be there.

"Hello, Mrs. Prince. How long have you been feeling sick?" John didn't waste time with the pleasantries.

She admitted to a day.

John asked her where she hurt, but she brushed him off. She insisted she didn't need to be there.

She sounded like the classic elderly person: stoic. It made them hard to trust. Live through World War II, lose a son in Vietnam, and nothing else hurts. "Are you in pain?" is answered with, "No, but I have a little tenderness." You need a concerned spouse to tattle on them. The patient might say "days," but I believe it when the spouse says "weeks."

Her story warranted another rectal exam. I just couldn't escape them. I slipped my gloved finger in and the tip collided with a firm mass. Cancer. A prime example of "Trust No One." The medicine doctor either had really short fingers, or didn't have her finger in the patient's butt when she had performed the rectal. I told John and he repeated the exam because he couldn't trust me either.

A mass this large and this low wouldn't be easily removable. She needed a diverting colostomy; in other words, she'd have to poop out of the side of her abdomen into a plastic bag. A completely obstructed bowel was life threatening.

"I'm too old for surgery," she whined. Her face became one squinty wrinkle. "Just let me die. You won't be able to cure me."

John argued otherwise. "If we don't relieve your obstruction now, you will be begging us for surgery in a couple of hours. This isn't something you can die a peaceful death from. At least let us do that for you."

"I don't know. Let me talk to my granddaughter. Have her come here."

Her granddaughter had disappeared. So, I started writing our consult note in the chart.

"C'mon, you're killing me," John said. "They're going to consult us another five times before you finish the note."

"You need to have some patience," I said. I bet he watched movies in fast-forward.

"I know," he said. "I wish I was more like our attending. He's always calm."

"That's a good lesson to learn. If you pester your daughter like you pester me, she's going to end up a nutcase." John had a tendency to grab things to show me the right, i.e., his "most efficient," way to do it. I hated that. My dad did that, too, and look what happened: I was a nutcase.

"I try, but I immediately forget. I can't stand wasted time."

Of course not, you're a surgeon. "I try to look at things through the five-year-retrospectroscope. These little inconveniences, like waiting for me to finish this note, or a scrub tech to get you an instrument, won't matter in five years."

"Sounds like a good idea. But if you don't hurry, it's going to be another five years before we eat. Why don't you finish that when her granddaughter gets here? We've only got another ten minutes of AFAT."

"AFAT?"

"Anesthesia Fuck Around Time. They're getting the next chole ready."

I gave up and John and I ran down to the cafeteria. I tried to find the food they couldn't screw up. An orange. Crackers. I was hungry and I was in a room full of food, but nothing looked edible. I felt like I was six years old and at a seafood restaurant. But, mom, don't they have hamburgers?

I found a complete hamburger wrapped in plastic. I turned it in my hands in disbelief. What were they thinking? The very place people get healed kills their healers with the food they serve. Now that's irony.

John ran off to do the cholecystectomy. I called the granddaughter of the bowel cancer lady. She said she lived fifteen minutes away.

She promptly arrived four hours later. Grandma didn't get her colostomy until midnight. Now she could poop into a bag attached to her abdomen. I used to tell friends that I couldn't join them dancing because I was afraid of breaking my colostomy bag. This year has put an end to that joke, at least for a while.

These patients were different from County patients. They didn't have complicated histories of drug abuse, untreated diabetes, and uncontrolled hypertension. County patients were significantly younger than the private ones with the same disease. The people with severe vascular disease at the county hospital were forty and fifty years old, whereas the privately insured were in their seventies. What a difference a healthy lifestyle makes.

By the time Sunday morning came, we had installed two

162

pacemakers, uninstalled two gallbladders, put in a diverting ostomy, and pulled out an appendix. In addition, I prepared a third pacemaker and evaluated a man with a GI (gastrointestinal) bleed. I was ready to go home and sleep the day away. On the drive home, I found myself wishing I had a 9 to 5 job, with weekends off. How could I become a Renaissance man? Leonardo Da Vinci hadn't spent all his time in the hospital.

Don't get me wrong; I loved operating. But did I have to enjoy curing so many hours of the week? I didn't do anything else. Most of my phone calls to Rachel were from the hospital—I spent my "one minute for myself" calling her. I could see why Corey thought having a family was so important while struggling through residency.

I wasn't ready for a family, but I did recognize how my brief conversations with her were little escapes into the realm of sanity. Maybe if she were out here it'd be a good thing, as long as she wasn't waiting for me.

At the same time, I wanted her to be a girlfriend, not just a source of decompression. I tried to avoid talking about work, which made her feel like I was holding out on her. I couldn't win.

I started another painting before I dozed off. This time it was a bunch of black fish with menacing teeth surrounding a red fish.

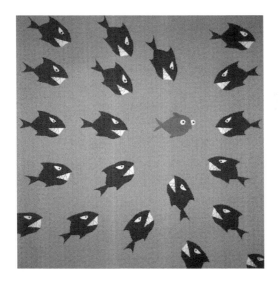

PART 3: THE COUNTY HOSPITAL AGAIN
Chapter 31

November. November! November 3rd is Day 146, 40% of 365. The clock does not stop.

Right back to County Hospital. The month-to-month schedule changed on the whim of Dr. Organ. The only thing set in stone (I hoped) was my vacation month—January.

The first thing I did when I returned was run to check my mailbox for the first time in two weeks. My paranoid side had convinced me that Dr. Organ sent me a list of menial tasks that were supposed to have been completed by yesterday.

Iaquinta, please present an anatomic description of the gubernaculum at the next conference.

Nope. But there was a letter from Dr. Irving, an apology for whacking Kendra. But it didn't say that. No, it was a generic letter written in the same passive, third-person point of view as medical journal articles. Tensions run high in the OR. Sometimes things happen that shouldn't happen. I wondered if Kendra got it before she left for vacation.

I returned to the subspecies service. (That's what we dubbed the subspecialty service—Urology, ENT, and Neurosurgery.) But, this time I'd be paired with Mark, rumored to be an early front-runner for Intern of the Year. Corey told me Mark knew more than most third-year residents.

Mark was almost ten years older than me and as many times balder. He lacked the overbite, but looked enough like Montgomery Burns from *The Simpsons* to make me giggle.

We were organized, reliable, and hard working. But, despite our efforts, we couldn't succeed. We couldn't cover the OR for a neurosurgery case, urology clinic, and ENT clinic simultaneously.

I drew the short straw: Neurosurgery clinic. Usually I am a fly on the wall. Dr. Blanchard knows his patients but likes me there to "hold hands." And with good reason—I'd want my hand held if my brain were going to be cut into.

I walked into clinic to find Dr. Blanchard decked out in magenta scrubs hollering into the phone. If the person receiving the berating could have seen his sissy pink scrubs, his yelling would have lost all effect.

"That doesn't sound like an operating room to me. I don't know what you are running down there, but it doesn't sound like an operating room." He shook the phone at no one. "See, I need nurses to schedule cases and move patients in and out of rooms. I need anesthesia to see patients. I need people to turn over the rooms. People just can't call in sick. Why are you doing this to me?"

That was his modus operandi. He tried to convince people that they personally insulted him by not having whatever he wanted done. He mistakenly assumed that they would be motivated by their overwhelming guilt.

Dr. Blanchard slammed down the phone.

"Good morning, Dr. Blanchard. I am going to help you in clinic this morning, but I have to go see a patient in the ER first. I'm on call and Mark's in the OR."

"Sal, I need you here to help me. This is not a neurosurgery service; if I have to get everything done myself then this is not a service. You are supposed to provide the service...TO ME."

"Okay." I didn't know what to do. I waited.

"Well, don't just stand there, go see that patient and get back here!"

I ran off to the ER.

Black netting masked the face of the restrained patient in the hall nearest the ER door. She must have tried to spit on the passersby, but the black bug net made it look like she was being hospitalized for being kinky. As I walked by she said, "She called me nuts. I like pecans, cashews, and walnuts. And these aren't even my real teeth."

I giggled as I walked into the doctor's workroom to find the patient's chart. The ER doc—the one that occasionally flipped around a butterfly knife and was always wearing a fishing vest with medical gadgetry jammed into the pockets—lectured the few residents in the room.

"When you get a patient that refuses your recommended treatment, like taking a medicine, don't just document it. Document what the patient says," he advised. "If you look through some of my notes you will see things like 'Go fuck yourself, you cocksucking motherfucker. I'm not taking that pill, I'm getting out of this fucking place.'

"That guy is the type of guy that will sue. He'll go home and realize he should have stayed at the hospital and taken the pill. Then, because of some complication, he decides to sue and you're screwed when you get to court because you didn't document exactly what happened.

"I've been saved from going to court because the patient changes his mind after he sees his statements documented. Every guy looks good with a new suit and their hair combed, but when he has to agree that he told me 'Fuck yourself, shithead, I'm getting out of here,' he's the one who looks like an idiot."

The rookies chuckled and eagerly nodded their heads in agreement.

It was exactly what I needed to hear on my way to see a drunken guy who had ripped out his Foley catheter. I cringed at that thought. The balloon inflates in the bladder so the catheter can't slip out, which meant he had pulled really hard as he yanked a balloon nearly the size of a Ping-Pong ball out of his penis.

Five occupied gurneys filled the room, but the stench of alcohol sweat gave my patient away. A white sheet partially covered the lower half of his scrawny body. Was he sleeping? His snarled gray hair hung down just far enough to make it hard to tell.

"Sir?" I leaned toward him.

"Whaaaaaaaat?" Yes, he was still drunk. Why did disheveled people have three days of scruff? Did this mean that three days ago he had been a clean-cut man, not an unkempt drunk?

"You need that catheter in. Why did you pull it out?"

"If I wanted the fucking thing in, I wouldn't have yanked it out."

"Well..." He had me there.

"My dick had better be all right or I'm going to sue you! I'm going to remember you. I'm going to make your life shit if my dick don't work." He pointed a gnarled finger with a dirty, split fingernail at me.

Doesn't work. You are going to make my life shit if your dick doesn't work.

"If you want your penis to work," I said, "then I suggest you do what I say. Leave this catheter in for four days so as the wound inside heals, it doesn't stricture. If it scars down without the Foley in, then you will need surgery so you can pee again."

He grumbled in agreement. "It better work or it's your ass."

No, it's your penis. The temptation to snap back was almost

166

irresistible.

I documented his threats and curses verbatim into the chart. It refreshed me to write naughty words in an "official" document.

That was my minute for myself. And actually one that I'd share with Rachel. She had enough medical knowledge to know to squirm and moan when I mentioned that the patient yanked the catheter out with the balloon up.

Chapter 32

We were back to having M&M conference at 7 a.m. and there weren't any extra observers. Dr. Organ had clearly won the battle while I'd been away.

Dr. Organ glowed; he looked like a dog about to be fed a porterhouse. Corey was no longer chief resident; John had taken his place. Dr. Organ had a fresh chief to sink his teeth into.

"John, what did you find in last night's ex-lap?" Dr. Organ asked. An ex-lap is an abdominal exploration.

"We found a fibrous band impinging a loop of small bowel that we broke down bluntly."

Dr. Organ interrupted, "Broken down bluntly? Sounds physical. Did you use a baseball bat?"

John didn't hesitate. "No, finger dissection." Cool as ice cream.

I smiled, but John didn't.

"John, what about this melanoma case from two days ago? Where do you think sentinel lymph node biopsy will be in five years?" He raised an eyebrow at John. When he does that, you know he is already skeptical of your answer, no matter what you say. He had a rebuttal ready.

"It will be here," John said. He knew to answer Dr. Organ with assured direct answers.

"Your confidence impresses me, but your knowledge base does not," Dr. Organ chuckled.

That made John smile. "Sentinel node is technically easy and well-tolerated by the patient. It will be here."

Dr. Organ's jabs didn't intimidate John, so he turned to weaker prey: me.

"Iaquinta." Dr. Organ turned his head to me.

I felt my back perspire. It's amazing how fast it can shoot out sweat when you are nervous. Dr. Organ grinned like a hungry tiger looking at a lame gazelle.

"The other day when we opened that abdomen full of pus, we didn't find an obvious source of infection. "Where do you think all that pus came from?"

His question referred to the woman we had taken to the OR

because of the way she looked. But that had been over a month ago. Unless he meant someone else's case and he thought I was with him.

He didn't give me any time to answer. "Common things are common. I would bet that it was from the appendix. More often than not I will be right. But, if you go looking for rare things, you will rarely be right."

He looked at me. "Where else could it be from?"

"I agree with you: the appendix."

"C'mon, where else could it be from? From the mouths of babes can come words of wisdom."

There were a few chuckles.

I fed off John's boldness. "I would rather remain silent and play the fool than open my mouth and remove all doubt." Touché. More chuckles. Evan loved it. So did I; I had just gotten away with smarting off to the big man. Yes!

"Oh, come on, now." He gave me a slow smile. Everyone looked at me.

"It could have been from a pelvic infection."

"No, I don't think it could have been. Her tubes looked perfect."

Fine, I'm proved the fool. You win.

He moved on to Franklin.

"Franklin," he said.

"Yee-ahh," Franklin replied. Everyone cringed at his slang.

Dr. Organ's brow wrinkled. "I don't understand why you lower yourself to that vernacular. All those years in medical school and you talk like the people who come into this place. You sound like a janitor. I know you think you are all cutesy, but you are a doctor."

Franklin sheepishly said, "Yes, sir."

The incident made Dr. Organ forget the question he was going to ask Franklin, so he went back to pimping John. That's what we call the needling questioning attendings use as both a form of education and verbal abuse.

That was more fuel to my Alzheimer's-theory fire. How many times was he going to say, "common things are common"? And why did he pick a case from a month ago when we were supposed to be

169

discussing the last week's cases?

On the way out of conference I asked John if Dr. Organ had been like that a few years ago.

"He doesn't have the brilliant edge he used to have, but he's still a sharp guy." John said.

The medical literature says that eighty percent of 80-year-olds have signs of dementia. Just how old was Dr. Organ?

Chapter 33

Breakfast was mandatory for me. Without it, I'd die. Every morning I had my Cinnamon Toast Crunch mixed with Rice Chex, or Lucky Charms mixed with Cheerios. That morning I missed breakfast, but didn't make the effort to stuff patient's graham crackers into my mouth because Dr. Blanchard was going to buy us lunch. I wanted to be hungry for a good, free meal. In hindsight, I'd never start 48 hours of straight call without breakfast again.

The morning started with a tonsillectomy—the bread and butter case of my future career. Hopefully Dr. Schmidt would let me do one side.

Dr. Schmidt was the county's seldom-seen otolaryngologist. He shared one thing in common with many of County patients: He had no lower front teeth. He used a bridge to hide the fact he lost them in a motorcycle accident. Otherwise he was a short, skinny white guy with expensive-looking wire glasses. He had a private facial plastics practice to which he devoted most of his time and thoughts.

He worked at County for his one day a week of community service. He had come to improve the life of a 27-year-old girl with recurrent tonsillitis. After she was intubated, Dr. Schmidt stuck a metal retractor into her mouth. It held her mouth open and the tongue down, giving us a great view of the tonsils.

"Watch me do the first side and I'll let you do the second." He grabbed the tonsil with a clamp and pulled it medially (toward the midline). He carved it from the surrounding tissue with the Bovie. I sucked the smoke for him. But then she started bleeding. Chronically infected tonsils are both rich in blood vessels and fall apart easily (vascular and friable). The endotracheal tube's inflatable cuff prevented the blood from going down the throat, which made it pool up in her mouth. The pooling blood in her mouth was very horror-movie-esque to me.

When he finished his side, he grabbed the sucker from me and suctioned her throat. Then, he handed me the instruments. "Just find the plane and dissect the tonsil off of it."

Sure. I grabbed the tonsil with the curved clamp. I retracted it from its fossa. Rip. The clamp pulled loose, tearing off a piece of tonsil. "Sorry."

"Just regrasp it and go."

It looked so easy until I tried it.

Dr. Schmidt let me struggle for a few minutes. I got most of the tonsil out, but he took over to control the bleeding.

It's hot in this surgical gown. It sure would feel nice to take off my gloves and mask and fan myself. Look at all that blood coming out of her mouth. Wasn't there a part in *The Shining* like this? Yeah, the blood poured out of the elevators.

Every pore in my body started sweating.

Wait a minute, I know what's happening. I'm getting vasovagal. All of my blood vessels are dilating. Soon I won't have enough blood volume to get up to my head. "Dr. Schmidt, I'm sorry, but I have to sit down."

He shook his head in disappointment. "I'm not sure you're going to make it in this field." He went back to cauterizing the bleeders.

Normally I'd vehemently protest such a perception, but I really needed to get to the stool.

Almost there.

I entered a new world, a black world. Silent. Peaceful. I drifted slowly, deep underwater. There was something down there. I could see the edges of unidentifiable objects dimly glowing a dark purple, glowing like those deep-sea fish that can phosphoresce.

Suddenly, hands were shaking my shoulders and people were calling my name. By the time I opened my eyes I was on a gurney heading out of the operating room. My gloves and mask had been ripped off. My gown was still on, but torn open. Sweat saturated my scrubs.

I called back to Dr. Schmidt "I'm sorry" as I got wheeled out of the room. I didn't get to see that disappointed look he always gives when he is inconvenienced.

The anesthetist told me, "Sit still on the gurney because the rails aren't up."

Come on. I know that. We say that to every patient, but we have the rails up.

I went to the recovery room as a patient.

The nurses wrapped a blood-pressure cuff around my arm, put EKG leads on my chest, a pulse oximeter on my thumb, and a nasal cannula to deliver oxygen on my nose. I was mostly normal; my heart rate was 42 beats a minute. Normal is 60 to 100.

"He's soaking," one nurse said.

"Look how pale he is," another observed.

For once I felt like the fallen alien I often pretended to be. They finished their prodding and offered me fruit juice. Hospitable creatures, I thought. Strange greeting practices. Once they were bored with me, they scattered off to other corners like dust bunnies from the broom.

I drank my juice and refused a blueberry muffin. Those things are loaded with fat.

Another one offered me a chocolate brownie.

I declined it.

"Typical male. You must be all right."

"I am just trying to watch my petite figure," I jested.

"I am getting the feeling you don't eat the types of food we're offering you," the skinny nurse hypothesized. "Do you want a banana?"

"Please."

I humbly ate my banana and finished my juice. My pit stop was over.

I called over to the nurses in my best disgruntled patient voice, "Give me some morphine. I'm in pain."

They looked at me skeptically.

"I was just kidding."

They nodded politely.

I sat up and pulled the EKG leads off.

"I guess you're leaving AMA," the nurse said. Against Medical Advice.

"Yep, back to work."

"You really should have the day off after something like this."

I laughed. I could just imagine the look on Dr. Organ's face if he heard I had left for the day. One of the on-call trauma team residents had gastroenteritis last month. She ended up sleeping in an empty ICU bed with an IV hooked up to her arm to replenish her fluids. No, you were either healthy enough to work or so sick you had to stay at the hospital. Either way, you belonged at the hospital.

"I'm on call today," I called back to her. As I walked away, I noticed how sweaty I was. Underwater World? Gross.

I went back into the OR. Dr. Schmidt had just finished.

"Sorry for passing out. What did I miss?"

"Well, when you walked away from the table I could tell you weren't going to make it to the chair so I backed into you and pinned you against the wall until the circulator grabbed you. You're lucky this didn't happen when you were the only surgeon. The patient was still bleeding when you left us."

Yikes. I hoped that would never happen again.

It probably happened because I didn't have breakfast. I was probably hypoglycemic.

That, and I am a big sissy. Ick, blood.

Chapter 34

The whole hospital pitied Mark and me. Everyone knew we were the only two on the specialty service and that we were getting pounded. An ER resident called me with a consult and she started with, "I'm sorry to call, but…" The ICU nurses had offered hugs to help console us after the loss of three patients within 24 hours from massive intracranial bleeds. I declined, mostly because I was afraid that the woman with the crew cut and giant biceps would squash the life out of me. I wished I could have taken the good parts of the three dying, brain-dead people to fix my broken patients up on the floor. Have a kidney. Here's a stomach. This bladder has a few miles on it, but it's in top working condition.

When I walked into the ICU that morning, I found Mark poised in front of a comatose patient with a drill in his hand. A nurse held the phone up to his ear while he stood in front of an unconscious twenty-year-old man lying in bed. Mark already had his sterile gloves on for whatever barbaric procedure he was about to undertake.

"What's going on? You need some help?" I asked when the nurse hung up the phone.

"Dr. Blanchard just told me how to put in a burr hole." Mark said comically.

"Where is he?" Dr. Blanchard, although difficult to reach, usually came in for procedures.

"He's operating at another hospital." Mark set the drill down and grabbed the scalpel. He made a small incision on the patient's scalp.

"What happened to him?" I nodded toward the intubated young man. His left pupil was dilated. The right was normal. I didn't see any evidence of head trauma.

"He's got a subdural abscess from his sinusitis." Mark set the scalpel down and lifted the drill. He rotated the crank to ensure the bit was on and aligned. "I got called from the ER about him a little while ago. They said he had a temp, a headache, and seemed groggy. The next thing I hear, they're calling a code. They intubated him and the scan shows a subdural abscess next to his sinusitis." He put the hand drill to the skull. After a few turns he was through the bone. Must have been a sharp bit. Or, maybe, it was just the fact that it was a young skull.

Mark pushed a catheter through the hole and gave it a little shove to penetrate the dura. Pus oozed out the top of the catheter.

"That smells feculent. I'll bet E. coli," Mark said.

I cringed away from the stench. About 10 milliliters of thick whitish-yellow pus came out. Just like Mark to say feculent when he should have said poop.

"Excuse me," a nurse interrupted. "Can one of you talk to his sister? She's on the phone."

"Sure," I offered. I talked to the sister; she said she'd be in shortly.

We waited for two days, but nobody came to visit him. I kept calling his sister back. When I finally got hold of her again, she told me he was a heroin addict and had been out of touch with the family.

I wondered what my own sister was up to. I couldn't have abandoned Jill in the hospital like that. When she had tried to commit suicide, I left medical school to go see her. But, now I hadn't talked to her in a couple of months. She rarely returned calls and I didn't try calling often. Maybe she'd been abandoned in some hospital, too.

*

Corey paged me that evening. He was at one of the private hospitals.

"Hey man, how's it going?"

"I'm all right, just a little beat up. All of my patients keep dying. Mark and I have been swamped." I had worked over 135 hours in the last week.

"Don't worry, once you're in ENT it will be smooth sailing," he said. "You know what the worst thing about every-other-night call is?"

"What?"

"You miss half the good cases." He giggled.

"Thanks, Corey."

"No problem, man. Hey, did you hear who I operated on?"

I didn't.

"Evan."

I hadn't seen Evan in two months. We were never at the same hospital.

Corey told me that Evan came to work complaining of abdominal pain. He had a history of a partial bowel obstruction after an accident a

176

few years ago. Corey talked about Evan like he was any patient. No preferential treatment.

"So, I watched him for a few hours in the ER and he progressed to a complete obstruction. He had a little internal hernia, but fortunately the bowel was healthy, after I untangled it.

"You know, it was strange. I couldn't help think, 'This is my friend' over and over as I operated."

"Sheesh, Corey. Your interns don't do what you want and you ex-lap them. I thought you were supposed to be the nice chief."

"I gave him the best of care. He's doing great. He'll go home tomorrow and get a couple of days to rest and hang out with his son."

"That's cool." Too bad it had taken an operation to get him some free time.

I wished my bowel were obstructed.

Chapter 35

I returned to have another patient die from yet another hemorrhagic stroke. What felt so unique and horrible to me happens all the time.

To declare someone brain dead, we first have to prove there isn't any brain function. The brain can be dead even if the heart is beating, which makes the situation confusing to most non-medical people.

The brain-death exam spooks me. And if it gave me goosebumps, there was no way I'd allow family members to be present. After they left, I warned the nurse what was about to happen. I didn't want her to let anyone visit, and I needed her help.

I started the examination with the eyes. I pulled the lids open and shone a bright light into them, looking for pupillary constriction. Then, I touched a cotton swab to the eye. That was the eerie part; he didn't blink. I hated eyeballs. Too squishy. After that, I checked the cough and gag reflexes. Then, I rubbed my knuckles firmly on his ribs to see if he responded to the pain. I imagined his ribs snapping under my hand.

He didn't respond to any of my tests. So we drew blood to evaluate the oxygen and carbon dioxide levels. They have to be normal or the exam wasn't valid.

I handed the blood sample to the nurse and asked her, "Can you make sure the lab does this STAT? Not in an hour or two."

"Start Taking Action Tomorrow," she replied.

"Huh?"

"That's what STAT means around here." She smiled.

"Go bust some skulls if you have to. Well, not skulls, I'm on neuro call."

I enjoyed working with her. Most of the ICU nurses had a sense of humor, and they were a thorough and trustworthy group. They had to be because their patients were so sick. Her blonde spiky hair accentuated her natural spunkiness. I always smiled when I saw her covering my patients. Okay, maybe I had a little crush on her.

The labs came back normal. I had the respiratory therapist stop the ventilator, after which we stepped back to wait ten minutes to see if the patient would take an unaided breath. Breathing is one of the brain's rudimentary functions. While we waited, Dr. Blanchard appeared in the background. He had a knack for showing up at just the right time. In a couple of minutes he would need to tell the family the patient was brain dead.

The respiratory therapist perched himself right in front of the patient's face. He gently stroked his goatee while staring intently at the patient, as if contemplating a chess move.

I leaned against the foot of the bed solely because my legs were tired of supporting me. But, the weight of my body transferred enough energy through the bed to make the patient's head nod.

"Ahhh!" The therapist jumped backward.

The nurse and Dr. Blanchard perked up.

"He moved," the therapist gasped.

I repositioned myself, causing the head to nod again. Everyone turned to look at me. I grinned. The therapist scowled, but the nurse and Dr. Blanchard saw the humor in the moment.

"I can't believe you guys can laugh," the therapist said.

"We are using laughter to displace our fears," I said smartly.

He said, "Right," but I knew he meant, "Fucker."

The patient made no effort to breathe during the entire ten minutes. We drew another blood sample to verify that the patient had supranormal levels of carbon dioxide in the blood. When the body senses excess carbon dioxide, it stimulates increased respirations—unless, of course, you're brain dead.

The man was dead. It was Friday and the man was dead.

When people die on Fridays it reminds me of my mom. When I was little, if my sister and I were fighting on a Friday my mom would say, "I hate it when my children kill each other on Friday; funerals ruin the weekend."

*

The only good thing about the day was that my little sister called for the first time in months. She sounded good. It was the first time in a long time that I heard her talk about living instead of wallowing in hate and self-pity. She had started taking classes at a community college and she was living in a rehab facility. She said she actually felt happy for the first time in years without using drugs. She told me "rehab is a great place to meet people!"

"Maybe I should check it out," I said.

Chapter 36

That night, on call, a man came in from a terrible car accident. He had been speeding down a city street (without his seatbelt on) and crashed into a telephone pole. The firefighters had used the Jaws of Life to get him out of the mangled car.

Someone on the rescue team took Polaroid photos of the accident and sent them with the patient to the ER. I have no idea why—maybe to quote him a repair estimate. If car damage indicated his chance of survival, this one predicted I-don't-think-so.

But we were going to try anyway.

His body didn't look that bad compared to the car. Sure, he had an open-skull fracture in which you could see a chunk of bone the size of a credit card slightly depressed on his forehead. And when the bleeding slowed down from the overlying gash, I could see the white edge of his broken skull.

The rest of his bruised face looked like a bloated eggplant. Chunks of windshield glass filled his right ear canal. Amazing how they flew in there. A little bit of gooey blood sat in the left ear canal, but no glass.

His right tibia poked out of the skin of his right shin ever so slightly and his foot leaned too far out to the side. I grimaced. No way could I have done orthopedics. Broken bones poking through skin rank second to squishy eyeballs. I always imagined the victim trying to use the broken limb. In this case if he got onto his feet his body would slump to the floor, ripping the skin and muscle away from the tibia. And that's what gave me the willies.

There was also some blood at his urethral meatus (the pee-hole), an indicator of a pelvic fracture. The trauma team leaves no stone unturned, no hole unprobed. So don't follow your mom's saying about always wearing a clean pair of underwear in case you go to the hospital in an emergency. They immediately cut your clothes off with a large scissors. So, wear your worst clothes whenever you go for a drive.

After we stabilized him, we brought him to the CT scanner. The depressed skull fracture didn't push into the brain. His brain looked normal. The CT also confirmed a pelvic fracture.

When we reevaluated him in the ICU, he didn't withdraw from pain. He didn't flinch when the medical student started a line on him. Even worse, the orthopedist set his tibial fractures with external pins without anesthesia. I was saying how close to brain dead he was when someone noticed on the CT scan that there was extra fluid around the aorta.

He had probably torn his aorta, the largest artery, the fixed stalk on which the heart "swings" in the chest. During a deceleration accident the heart can slam forward as the body stops, causing the aorta to rip.

We brought him back downstairs for an aortogram, and sure enough, he had a tear in the posterior descending aorta about five centimeters long. That meant he would have to be transferred to a nearby hospital, since County Hospital didn't have a cardiac bypass machine.

The trauma team wanted the blessing of Dr. Blanchard to send the patient to another hospital. In other words, they wanted him to say the patient was neurologically stable for transfer. "Brain dead" seemed stable to me. Couldn't be more stable than dead.

Dr. Blanchard said, "The only reason to repair that aorta is to save the organs for donation." Then he asked, "Why are you going to transfer him to get his repair anyway?"

"They don't do aortic repairs here."

"I've got 'they' right here in my car with me," he said. "Why don't you let the trauma chief tell us what's going on?"

By a stroke of bad luck, Dr. Fagan, the vascular surgeon, was in Blanchard's car. Despite not having a bypass machine, he felt that he could quickly repair the aorta. When the trauma chief hung up the phone I apologized to him for the change of events. His tired face sank even closer to the ground when he learned he was going to be up all night performing Mission Impossible.

While too many of us stood around as the patient was being prepared for the OR, one of the junior residents said to me, "This is what we call a bad save. Have you heard of that?"

I thought it sounded self-explanatory.

But he explained anyway. "Medicine has progressed to the point where we can keep almost anyone alive. The problem is that we haven't learned how to choose when to use these modalities. There isn't a good outcome for this young man." He talked like a robot, a common behavior among residents with a couple years under their belt. Beaten into monotony. I've one-upped them, though: I've been monotonous since the sixth grade.

"I know. The best case scenario looks like a vegetable."

"A short-lived vegetable. But we will spend tens of thousands guaranteeing it."

Later that night, I met the patient's sister. She insisted that he must have been run off the road because he was such a good driver. They were going to look for clues at the accident scene. Maybe someone had seen who was responsible. I couldn't tell her that her brother's blood alcohol level was over three times the legal limit due to the health information privacy laws. He was lucky he hadn't killed anyone else.

I struggled to keep my mouth shut. I wanted to set her straight. Misconceptions were not allowed. There would be no false laying of blame on my shift.

He made it through the six-hour operation. Actually, his brainstem made it through the operation. His only sign of life consisted of occasional spontaneous respirations.

Why Dr. Fagan bothered I didn't know. He hadn't come in that day to help the woman with the bowel obstruction, so why had he come in at midnight to perform such a futile case?

Hubris must have been involved. But, there was something more. Many physicians thought that the goal was to restore not the quality of life but the quantity of life.

It takes a boatload of deep thoughts to figure out what our society should do with medically futile situations. Such thinking was not going to happen at 5 a.m. Let's just say that my brain was in the shallow end with floaties on. But the good thing about 5 a.m. in Oakland is that it is 8 a.m. in New York city. This allowed my ambitious, early-rising friend to write me for free medical advice. The type of advice I could answer, the type of advice only he would ask.

A brief excerpt:

> Incidentally, is there any drug that can turbocharge your metabolism to such an extent that your body feeds upon its own muscle mass? And if so, what would be the best thing to eat to counteract this effect, particularly if there were no plant or wild life? Human flesh would suffice.
>
> Also, is there any part of the human body, specifically, that a person could consume and feel instantly stronger, such as adrenal glands or

something to that effect... Specific organs would be useful. Even if it's quite a stretch, any information would be useful.

Oh yeah, can the human jaw generate enough force to bite through a human skull?

Please say no...

I am not insane.

Do you think it's possible to get floor plans to the White House?

I'll explain more later.

What do you know about medicinal treatments for radiation poisoning? Is there such a thing?

I might be from Wisconsin, but I wasn't buddies with Jeffrey Dahmer or Ed Gein. This consultation was for a zombie screenplay.

Too bad attendings don't ask questions this good. I gave him my best answers. I felt that the thyroid glands and the adrenals would be the most appropriate zombie delicacies.

Then I thanked him for assuring that my years of studying weren't going to waste.

Chapter 37

A couple of days before Thanksgiving my mom called to tell me that my sister ran away from rehab once again. The story this time was that a urine test turned up positive for morphine derivative, but she insisted that she was not using drugs. She wanted a blood test done to prove her innocence but they wouldn't do it. She thought that the positive test was due to the cough syrup she was taking.

So she got mad and left.

I would like to believe her. Maybe the offending chemical was the dextromethorphan in an over-the-counter cough syrup. Hardly the thing to get a rush off of if you're used to the real deal. But the story sounded too much like the stories of County Hospital.

Of course, I didn't get an answer, because she didn't call. And if we did talk, I wouldn't ask. That would make me just another one of her bad guys. Instead, we would have talked about music and movies and anything else that skirted around the real issues.

I figured with my mom and the counselors being the bad guys, she needed someone she could talk to without arguing. She already knew what she was doing wrong. It was up to her to quit, just as the woman with the neck abscess had said. So, I stayed her supportive brother. I did my best to not enable her while at the same time not alienating her. My biggest fear was that if she thought she was alone, she might attempt suicide again.

*

Rachel visited for the Thanksgiving Day weekend.

We made homemade butter rolls to bring to John's house. I didn't scrape the bowl. Well, not too obsessively.

The weekend passed effortlessly. After she left I found a note that told me how she felt.

See ya later, Salsa. Wish I didn't have to go and I wish you weren't an intern and I weren't a 2nd year and you weren't in Oakland and me in Madison...or at least one of each of those last two. Love, Rachel.

Maybe just the last one.

Chapter 38

The next morning I returned to the trenches. I stopped by the room of a young man recovering from a small abscess.

"I need better pain control. I need methadone more than once a day. I had a five hundred dollar a day habit before I came into here. I got myself loaded and then I took 150 mg of methadone before coming to the hospital the other night. The stuff you're giving me now doesn't touch me."

I thought about this a second. "How did you afford 500 dollars a day?"

"I became a drug dealer."

Logically. Crap, how did my sister pay for drugs?

"I didn't even want to start using drugs, but I broke my ankle in fourteen places and haven't had it repaired yet," he pointed to his right ankle. "See, I was bit by this Rottweiler and it shoved me off the second floor of a building. I broke my ankle when I hit the ground. It looked like this." He gestured with his hand, demonstrating his foot hanging off at a ninety-degree angle to the side.

"Ihhahhh." Orthopedic injury. Ick.

"Yeah, and I didn't get the surgery yet. I started using to treat the pain."

"Okay, let me see what I can do to help you." First, we need to get you off drugs. Then, we need to teach you drugs are bad. And dirty needles are worse. Then, we need to fix your ankle...

"I need that methadone twice a day," he said. "Otherwise by night I need to use. A guy stopped by my room last night with some heroin, but I decided I didn't want it. Shooting drugs got me this infection in the first place. That's not what I wanted. I don't want to be a drug user."

I commended him while writing the methadone order. Who needs candy-stripers when there are heroin-stripers? And why did a Rottweiler push him off the second floor of a building? The detective wanted answers.

As I walked down the hallway I realized that the internship lost its mystique. His crazy story didn't excite me; it saddened me. Life's not supposed to be that messed up. Not my life anyway. I realized that everyone who really mattered to me was over a thousand miles away. What I really needed was that darned teleporter so that I could visit

Rachel, my mom, and my old friends. I concentrated extra hard, but the farthest I got was to the next patient's room.

Then, as an added insult, when I checked my mailbox I had a letter from Dr. Organ. The very thing Corey warned me about. I hoped for tickets to Hawaii as I unfolded the flap. Nope. He assigned me the task of giving a 5-minute presentation on aortic balloon pumps.

Later that evening, after seeing a young Hispanic woman that would never wake up out of her coma, I decided to use my "one minute" to call Rachel and decompress.

I didn't expect her to confess to me that the boy next door gave her a backrub. She and her roommate had won backrubs from the neighbors for beating them in a board game. But then she confessed that they cheated to win.

"You cheated to win?" My girlfriend cheats at board games?

"Yeah, but the backrub was lousy."

Like that meant it didn't count?

"Don't you know that 95% of backrubs lead to sex and the other five percent lead to people lying about not having sex after getting their backrub?"

She laughed.

Maybe she laughed a little too hard. Hmmm.

"So, did you have sex or not?"

"No, of course not." She laughed again.

"So you're one of the liars," I hollered.

She just laughed more.

"I know you're just laughing to put off answering."

"Okay, okay, I had sex with the neighbor boy."

"I know what you're doing. You're telling me the truth but passing it off as a joke to clear your conscience. This way when I really find out you can tell me you told me so."

She just kept laughing. Apparently this breach in our monogamous relationship was merely a joke.

186

Chapter 39

December and back on the Green Team. This time with John as chief.

*

That evening I found out that the guy whose leg Corey and I had amputated three months ago had died. I wasn't too surprised. He had so many other health problems. About thirty percent of people who need amputations die within one year of them.

But he was the only non-comatose patient I knew of who had died after discharge from my service. At least I had never come down on him for smoking cigarettes in his room.

It made me realize that my successes would merely be brief delays for the inevitable. We really weren't in control; no matter how hard we tried.

Maybe someday I could have a sign made up to hang in my waiting room that says, "If you are my patient, you will die. But, if you aren't my patient, you'll die too, maybe faster." That sign, along with a small aquarium, ought to put people at ease.

Chapter 40

I would have rather yanked out my toenails with pliers than give my presentation that morning before Grand Rounds. The last time I had to do a public presentation I got so nervous that my voice started throwing wild pitches.

My fear of public scrutiny came from my days of forced piano lessons. I hated piano. To this day, I blame my mom for ruining my basketball career. If only she would have let me go to Saturday morning basketball with my friends instead of those stupid lessons. I don't see Nike looking for the next Liberace to wear their shoes.

I used to be more courageous. I loved being in school plays back in first and second grade. I was Rumplestiltskin. I was the stranger who came to town in "Stone Soup." I was a star. I was huge. I was Someone. But then, things changed.

My fourth grade piano recital. I remember it clearly: It was a spring day and I was wearing a stupid yellow sweater, which I had liked until that day. My family and I sat in the tenth row, almost all the way back. It sure seemed like there were a lot of people there. While the other kids played, the back of a few dozen heads morphed into thousands of heads. I didn't want thousands looking at me. My piano teacher announced I was going to play Für Elise. Or so she thought.

Instead I went up to the piano. Sat down. Put my hands on the keys. Boy, there are a lot of people looking at me. And there must be twice as many eyes as people! Wasn't there anything else to look at? Is that a squirrel outside? Hey everyone! Put your fingers in your ears and look at the squirrel. Shoot, I can't move my fingers. Why don't my fingers work? What was I going to play anyway if my fingers did work?

It was like someone had partially thawed a Neanderthal and set him at the piano. I only knew one thing: Oog.

Suddenly, I remembered how to cry. So I did. I stood up, put my head down, and shuffled out of the room. The entire place sat in silence. But for all I knew they were looking at that squirrel with fingers in their ears, because I didn't dare look up.

Weeks later, I found the pictures my dad had taken of me sitting frozen at the piano and then walking out of the room. Why had he taken pictures of my worst moment? Maybe Proud Dad wanted photographic evidence of his Going-To-Be-Great Son's only failure. I discreetly lost those pictures in the garage, somewhere near the garbage cans. I think they were accidentally ripped in half, too.

I never recovered. When I graduated from eighth grade I was one of the "honored" kids. My mom said that I could go on to be valedictorian of the high school.

"Would I have to speak at graduation?"

"Yes, but so does the salutatorian, the second-place person," she told me.

"Well, then I'll graduate third."

"That's good enough for me."

I graduated third in my class.

I was too scared to take a speech class in high school, and I avoided speeches in college. I was rarely forced to speak in public; the science curriculum doesn't lend itself to many student talks. I discovered I could partially revert back to my frozen Neanderthal state for presentations. My fingers got so cold that my nails turned purple and I say "oog" a lot.

I punctuated the hours before my aortic balloon pump presentation with numerous trips to the bathroom. It gave me a chance to sit and practice my talk.

I attempted to displace anxiety with elaborate fantasy. I wished that I could walk to the front of the room and say, "A discussion of balloon pumps would be a gross misuse of your time. Instead, Dr. Organ will sing the tale of Daedelus and Icarus as if it were a classic Italian opera. I will be acting the part of Daedelus." Everyone would look at me in disbelief as I jerked my head to Dr. Organ, spread my arms like wings, and said, "Ah one, two, three, four."

Instead, I distracted my audience with overheads. I looked up once during the five minutes and realized I didn't really want to look at them. Doctors are ugly, remember? As I raced through it, I realized that they actually want to hear what I had to say. If they were going to scrutinize anything it would be the information, not my delivery of it. I didn't matter. I was just the transfer medium. Those white eyes, two per head, weren't even looking at me; they were looking at the overheads.

My voice didn't crack. And when I finished I felt good, not just relieved. Something in me had changed. It was a year of sink or swim, and I performed swimmingly.

Afterwards, when I was in the hallway, one of the senior residents praised me. "Easy to follow and straight to the point."

That was the first time someone had ever said something like that. I was used to hearing people say, "You shouldn't be so nervous. It's no big deal." This, to me, was the equivalent of a suicidal patient seeing a psychiatrist and having the shrink say, "You shouldn't be so depressed, life is good. Now run along."

Dr. Mad-doodler said to me, "Excellent presentation this morning. And great tie."

YES! Of course, great presentation. Undoubtedly great tie.

Corey threw a wet blanket on me when he informed me that I'd have to do another presentation. Dr. Organ tapped the interns twice a year. Hadn't I proven enough? I'd rather work a fifty-hour shift without breakfast than present again.

They gave me a medical student as a reward. Some poor sap wanted to rotate at County Hospital. What perfect timing. I didn't enjoy waking up at four a.m. to round. But, now I had help. I had my very own human to boss around. To pimp. To corrupt. To embitter.

My minion proved to be both eager and competent. He rounded on four patients every morning, which saved me a half-hour. And I could send him in on the boring cases to be a human retractor so I could get work done on the floor during the day.

But most of all, I enjoyed the company. I needed someone to harass; someone to be the butt of my bad jokes without worrying about bruised ego repercussions. One morning he screwed up an order and I told him, "Well, you can only fail once for the day. I guess you got it out of the way early. Good job." Then for the rest of the day, every time he made a mistake I said, "Don't worry about it, you already failed for the day." John overheard me once and pulled me aside to say I shouldn't be so mean to the med student. But while the student may not have understood my jokes, he always grinned, so I thought he understood it was all in fun. I guess I'd see on my evaluation.

His first name was Hay. What a boon. People aren't named Hay in Wisconsin, animal food is. I could say, "Hey, did you get the labs on your patients?" and it sounded like I was addressing him. He was one of the rare exceptions where I remembered someone's name the first time I heard it. That says a lot, because I could meet a good-looking woman and have a great conversation and then realize I couldn't remember her name.

I told Hay that he needed to change his last name to You. Even

John joined in on that joke.

I also discovered that I enjoyed teaching. I liked to ask questions to make him think. I didn't care if someone couldn't memorize everything from a text, but if they couldn't think logically, it disappointed me. Hay could think.

Chapter 41

The orthopedists admitted a patient from the emergency room they wanted to transfer to our service. John asked me to go see him. When the "orthopods" came to the floor I was reading the chart.

"So what did you think?" the tall one with a crew cut asked.

"I don't know; didn't see him yet," I said. "I was just reading the chart to see what was going on."

"That's not a bad idea. But let's go look at that leg." He was still wearing those big plastic booties that they wear in the OR to protect their legs and shoes from blood.

"Reminds me of that joke," I said.

"What joke?"

"How do you hide a hundred dollars from an orthopod? Put it in the chart."

"Yeah, yeah." He already heard that one. "How do you keep a secret from a general surgeon?"

"How?"

"Tell it to his family."

That's a good one.

The guy had spilled boiling water on his lower leg. To make the situation worse, he had diabetic peripheral nerve disease, so he couldn't feel the water scalding him. Therefore, he didn't urgently remove his pants and cool the wound. He had a third-degree burn covering most of his lower leg. The skin on top of his toes and foot had sloughed off. Other parts looked like Freddy Krueger's face. He didn't have any pain because he had burnt his nerves to death.

I called John to tell him about the patient. He told me to admit him to our service. "That just shows how dumb those orthopods are," he said. "They were suckered by the ER into admitting a patient who doesn't have a single orthopedic issue. Get down to the OR right now and I'll let you do a cool case." John hung up.

I loved these little rivalries. We were all surgeons; the only thing that separated us was what we operated on. I guess that was enough. I think that if you were to draw a line down the middle of a crowded room it wouldn't take long before each side would claim the other side was for losers. Isn't that what state lines were? Why did all the trees in

Wisconsin lean south? Because Illinois sucks.

Yeah, there's something healthy about that. Even necessary. Right?

When I got into the elevator I joined a woman who was talking on her cell phone. She said, "He went with his grandpa to the horse track. He's only four so I thought he'd have fun seeing the horses. When he came home I asked if he had fun with grandpa and he said 'Yes.' Then, I asked if he learned anything and he put his hand in the air and yelled, 'Go fucking five.'" The woman shook her fist in the air, laughing.

"He was so darn cute while doing it I couldn't help but laugh," she continued.

Then the door opened and she went her way. Those twenty seconds were a perfect rebuttal to Corey's argument to always take the stairs. And I still had 40 seconds left of my "one minute."

*

John provided me my operative highlight of the year: my first solo laparoscopic appendectomy. A 20-year-old girl came in the night before for what I thought looked like appendicitis. She had pain in the right spot, a little bit of a temperature, and an elevated white count. But, the resident who saw her wasn't sure, and not being the type to risk losing a quarter to John, she chose to observe her. That resident's hesitation became my perfect opportunity.

John somehow convinced Dr. Roland, the youngest (and therefore most open-minded) attending, to let us start the case and only scrub in if there were any difficulties. Roland agreed; he was obviously confident with John's abilities.

I did an end zone dance on the way to the OR. A slender girl with a virgin abdomen! That meant no thick fat and no scar tissue left over from previous surgery.

As soon as the patient was "tubed," John began rushing me. "C'mon, c'mon, c'mon. Let's get this done before Roland comes and takes this case away from you." Other people might mistake his encouragement for badgering. But if John felt comfortable with a case, he didn't want an attending there. They only slowed things down. John had already developed his own "more efficient" style.

I stabbed the skin just below her umbilicus. Then, I spread the fascia open with a hemostat. John put in a clamp and grabbed the inside stump of the belly button and pulled up.

"Alright, put the Veress needle in, quit holding up the case."

The Veress needle is a skinny metal needle about six inches long that you stick into the abdominal cavity. Once it is in, you hook up the tube that blows carbon dioxide into the abdomen. I didn't like the idea of bluntly jabbing a needle into the abdomen without being able to see where it was going. There are too many horror stories of surgeons puncturing the bowel. But that didn't stop me.

I felt it pop through one layer.

"You should feel it pop through two layers," John said. Did he hear the first pop?

I pushed harder and felt the second pop. "All right."

John attached a syringe to the end of the needle and aspirated. Some air came back. That meant that we were in the abdominal cavity, or the bowel. We hooked up the gas and let it flow in. It flowed in easily at low pressure; that meant we were in the abdominal cavity.

In about two minutes the girl's abdomen bloated like a balloon. Just like Tom Cat in the cartoons.

John pulled out the Veress needle. "Put the 10 mm port in."

The scrub tech handed me what looked like an oversized meat thermometer, or maybe a medieval torture device. It was dull metal rod about one centimeter in diameter with a handle at one end and a menacing point at the other. It would really make the spies talk.

Dr. Roland entered the OR. With his mask on, he didn't look much older than Hay. Black hair poked out from under his surgeon's cap and his oversized glasses reminded me of Buddy Holly. I think he wore them to protect himself from splashes during trauma cases rather than a hipster fashion statement.

I once overheard him tell some residents that every patient that ever said to him, "I am going to die," did. You have to watch what you say to people.

He came to check up on us. "Aren't you guys done yet? I know you wanted to be done way before I ever came down."

John laughed as if it were a joke. He didn't deny it. We all knew he would be lying.

"Nice shave job," Dr. Roland said. The patient had a little peach fuzz on her belly below her umbilicus.

"I didn't want it to come back thicker," John replied.

"You're not concerned about infection?"

"No, in fact, you have a higher chance of infection if you shave just before the case. There are numerous articles to support it."

Roland laughed. He was just giving John a hard time. A freshly-shaved abdomen does have a higher risk of post-operative wound infection. But almost all County surgeons, including Roland, shave the abdomen before an operation to get the hair out of the way.

I put the torture spike into the hole I made under her belly button and started to push very carefully. I used my other hand as a brake.

"Makes you kind of nervous, doesn't it?" Roland said. "Don't like pushing such a sharp instrument toward the bowel?"

Of course it made me nervous, I couldn't see where it was going. Didn't he know I'd never done this before? Was he trying to make me anxious?

"I hate those things," he confessed. "This is the worst laparoscopic set I think they make. I like the disposable port system."

I felt the peritoneum pop. "There."

"Let me see that," John said grabbing it away. He wiggled the port around, pulled it out some, and pushed it back in. "Well, get the camera, don't just sit there all day."

"Camera."

"The camera isn't here yet," the scrub tech said. "Jackson was supposed to have put it in the sterilizer an hour ago, but when I came back from lunch he hadn't done it."

"What!" Roland hollered. "There must be another camera somewhere. Get it."

"There aren't any sterile ones."

"How long is it going to be?" John asked.

"About ten minutes," the circulating assistant answered.

"Ten minutes! That's ridiculous. We have a patient under anesthesia. How could you let a case start if the instruments aren't even here?" Roland asked.

"I thought it would take longer to get in," the circulator replied.

"Not only does the patient have increased anesthesia time, but it is costing one hundred dollars a minute just to have her in here. And that doesn't count our fees." Roland headed out the door. He needed to find a scope or someone to yell at, whichever was easier.

"The OR is a hundred dollars a minute?" Hay repeated.

John nodded yes.

"Boy, I got to get me in the OR leasing business," the scrub tech said.

"Just one is all you would need," John said.

Roland came back in empty handed. "I can't believe this. It is just starting its second rinse cycle." It sounded like laundry.

"Just grab it now," I kidded, "we're going to get it dirty anyway."

"Hey, no cutting corners." The circulator missed my joke.

John grabbed the port. "Why don't you try to look through there and do the surgery? Then we won't need the camera."

"Yeah," I agreed, "a true surgeon needs no eyes."

"Geez, look at this," John said, pointing to the wound. "I can see it granulating in. What's taking so long?" Granulation is a stage of the wound healing process.

Dr. Roland ran around with his arms in the air complaining for a few minutes. Then he went out into the hall and did it some more. Finally, he returned with the camera.

We hooked it up to the TV monitors. I put the camera into the abdominal port. We saw a normal-appearing uterus. A normal ovary. The large bowel.

"Move in," John ordered.

I advanced the camera. We could see a little bit of pus overlying the viscera.

"Aha," he said.

I angled the camera. The inflamed appendix came into view. Time for an appendectomy.

"All right, you have fifteen minutes before I scrub in," Roland warned.

Please don't let him scrub in, I prayed. I can do this. This isn't public speaking; this is my hands. I trust my hands. They'll get the job done.

196

We jabbed two more torture spikes into her abdomen. John put in a grasper to hold the appendix up through the superior port. I put one through the lower port to help him get a good hold of the appendix.

"Stapler," John called.

"Wait," Roland said. "Aren't you going to make a hole in the mesentery for the stapler?"

"No, I just take everything in one bite," John said. "It saves time."

"I like to take it in two staples. Put a hole between the appendix and the mesentery."

That's why John wanted to be done before Dr. Roland showed up. Too late. I grabbed a small pointed grasper and put it through the mesentery next to the appendix. I watched every move my hands made on the television monitor. It was a video game of sorts and I was a Tetris Master. I wished my mom could be there to see that my Nintendo years didn't go to waste.

"Make the hole a little bigger," Roland ordered.

"Eight minutes," Hay said. Apparently the atmosphere was lax enough that the med student could harass me. I took that as a compliment.

"Shut up." I whispered. Maybe Roland would lose track of time.

I made the hole and called for the stapler. The stapler has pincers like a wrench. I grasped the mesentery holding the appendix to the colon and clamped down on it. John made me rotate it so we could see what it was pinching on all sides. Nobody wanted to get the colon. I activated the stapler and it shot three rows of overlapping staples down the length of the pinchers. Then a blade slid down the inside of the pinchers and cut the specimen between the rows of staples. Very innovative.

"Reload," John said.

"Reload," the scrub tech said, looking at the circulator.

"I have to go get one."

"Come on! We just said we're taking it in two staples," Dr. Roland said. The circulator ran out of the room. "This place is a comedy. I am getting sick of it."

"Four minutes," Hay said.

I shot Hay a glare.

"I'm not even going to get lunch, this thing has been delayed so long," John complained.

The circulator returned. "This is all we have left." He set two reloads on the table.

Roland picked up one. "This is the wrong type," he complained. "It won't work for this type of stapler." He picked up the second one. "And this one doesn't have enough staples."

"Let's just use that one anyway," John suggested.

"Well, I want something more," Roland said. "Maybe you could tie it off."

"We could use the Endo-loop," John offered.

"Okay," Roland agreed. "I am going to scrub in if you can't get this on."

Not if I could help it. It was just another video game, and I had Pac-man fever. If I could save The Princess, I could lasso a lousy appendix.

I stapled off the bottom of the appendix. That left John hanging onto it in his clamp. I put in the endo-bag, which is a tiny bag on a purse string. John manipulated the amputated appendix into the bag and I pulled it out of the abdomen.

What looked so menacing on the TV screen was only the size of a ten-year-old's pinky finger. A mildly inflamed pinky finger.

"She's cured!" I exclaimed.

"Yeah, you saved her life." John sighed. "Now let's hurry up and tie off this stump and get some lunch."

I held the loop with the pinchers and, like a tiny cowboy, lassoed the appendiceal stump. I cinched the knot down and tied it. There was no chance for stool to leak into the abdominal cavity.

We took one last look around and then pulled out the instruments and ports. As the gas rushed out of the wounds, it made a pth pth pthhhhh noise.

"Geeeeeez," John said looking at me.

"Uh, excuse me."

No surgeon can resist the chance to make the abdominal-cavity-decompressing-fart joke.

And that was my first laparoscopic surgery as a surgeon. Definitely the highlight of the year.

*

When I got home I was so fatigued that I could barely drag myself up the stairs. To make things worse, they seemed to go on forever.

Then, I couldn't figure out why my key wouldn't open my door. I just wanted to go to bed.

"Who's there? Who is it?" A voice cracked from inside. I first wondered who was in my apartment, but fractions of a second later realized it was not my apartment.

I realized my folly and scampered back to the stairwell to my floor. I didn't hear the door open behind me. She probably thought I was the Grim Reaper and didn't dare open the door.

I didn't know a single tenant in my building. I had only seen the girl who parked in the spot next to mine once since I had moved in. I was the ghost of the building and I just scared the bejesus out of the woman upstairs.

Chapter 42

In clinic, I saw a man for a follow-up exam. He had the look of a Midwesterner. His flannel shirt was tucked in over his belly and a green baseball cap (sans John Deere logo) covered his bald head. He had been discharged from the hospital a week earlier after being treated for alcoholic pancreatitis. He had just kicked a heavy heroin habit, but still drank.

Quitting heroin and keeping a follow-up appointment both signified he truly cared about his health. I took the time to congratulate him for quitting narcotics, but warned him that that the alcohol had to go. He dodged a bullet with the pancreatitis but it could happen again. I asked him if he was still in pain.

"It hurts everyday. I have been using those pain pills, but they don't do much." He took off his hat as I sat down. "I was trying to only take them twice a day, but I need them three times."

"Are you drinking?" I asked. I used to be timid when I asked people their drug and alcohol habits, but this hospital had cured me of that. I already knew the answer—or someone had just spilled a drink on him.

He ran a hand across his bald scalp as he admitted that he was down to two fifths per day.

I shook my head slightly.

"I can't quit cold turkey. I have to go down slow, like I did with the heroin. My doctor told me that if I quit I could go into seizures and die."

I agreed and encouraged him to keep it up.

"I am," he said. "Just a month ago I was drinking a few pints a day. You wouldn't believe how much I've cut back."

Not being a drinker, I needed to figure out what fifths were. Ssince when do we divide anything by five? Couldn't we all go metric?

"When can I get the surgery to cure this pain?" he asked. "I think if my pain were cured I could focus more on quitting. It might not make sense to you in a science way, but drinking actually helps the pain."

His gallbladder indeed had stones. He was on the list to get it removed. But that might not cure his pain and I told him as much.

John walked by to see what was taking me so long. I quickly filled him in. But, John wasn't interested in prioritizing his cholecystectomy.

He could smell the alcohol. But he did take a second to poke his head through the curtain.

"You need to quit drinking, and then we can do the surgery," John said to him. "Have him come back when he has cut down," he said to me before walking away.

I asked the patient if he could be off alcohol in four weeks.

"You treat me like a person. A lot of 'em just come in here and talk to me like I'm a dog off the fucking street. I am going to quit."

I asked what made him decide. Maybe it was something I could transfer to my sister.

"I realized it would kill me."

I didn't see how that was a revelation. He clarified that he always knew it, but didn't care. So, I dug a little deeper and asked what really changed his mind.

He looked away. "When I had to clean my dad's brains off the wall."

"Whoa. I'm sorry." Probably should have left that stone unturned.

"A year ago, right before Christmas, 2:05 p.m. I walked into the room and BAM!" His eyes started watering.

The guy deserved to be a human. He was one, just in a lousy place.

"I've seen the way it's torn up my family and I'm not going to repeat that." His eyes started flowing.

I grabbed him a box of tissues. "Well, then you're going to do it."

"Thanks. Now let me get out of here before I make a scene."

Everything depends on perspective, not just my mom's busy day. Despite everyone knowing drugs and alcohol could kill him, it didn't matter until he realized they actually would kill him. And it took witnessing his dad commit suicide to drive that message home. How could I do the same for my sister and still keep my cerebellum inside my skull?

*

I bumped into the Dark Lord on my way out of the surgery library.

"How are you doing?" Dr. Organ asked.

I immediately felt a little nervous. It didn't make sense, but does it ever? "Pretty good. How are you?" I started grinning. That's me, The Grinning Fool. I grin when things are horrible, I grin when under pressure. Whereas most people have a whole repertoire of emotions and responses, I just grin. When my high-school principal questioned me about blowing off a firecracker during lunch, I just grinned. He told me I was acting guilty. My response? I grinned. What an ignorant fool he was. I wasn't the type to blow off firecrackers in school. And, if I were to blow them off, I wouldn't stand so close that a piece of shrapnel would cut my neck.

"Oh, I'm fine," Dr. Organ said. What are you up to?"

"I'm just borrowing this book so I can read up on a few topics if I have time on call tonight."

"You know, I have the new copy of Sabiston if you want to borrow it. Why don't you come down to my office?"

"Okay." As if I had a choice.

We were in his office and he was pulling a large book off his shelves when it came.

"Are you sure you want to go into otolaryngology?" he asked.

"Pretty sure." Time to play the game. Dr. Organ hated the gray zone. If given free reign in a consequence-free environment, I am sure I could have driven him mad with ambivalence.

"That doesn't sound 100% to me."

"It is hard to be 100% about something that I have never done. I suppose I won't really know until I do the residency."

That's how it is. That's the piece of information Rachel is missing. I couldn't predict how I'd feel about anything a year from now except cheeseburgers and oxygen. Emotions didn't follow the same straightforward trajectories of physics equation. I could tell you where a car will be 7 hours from now if it is moving north at 55 mph, but I can't tell you if the driver will actually be enjoying the drive.

"But why ENT?" Dr. Organ brought my attention back to him.

"The head and neck is the best anatomy of the body. Complex, compact, I like the precision and fine detail. It's an art." And there's no butthole to stick a finger into!

"Are you sure otolaryngology is the best way to get to do head and neck surgery?" He implied that some general surgeons did fellowships to learn some head and neck cases.

202

"Pretty sure. Every aspect of ENT interests me." Strangely, I found his subtle offer to be tortured for another four years in his program slightly flattering.

"I am going to have to call the director at your medical school and tell him he made a mistake. You should be a general surgeon," Dr. Organ kidded.

After I got out into the hallway, I realized I hadn't lived out my fantasy. When Dr. Organ requested, "Join me and I'll complete your training," I should have replied, "I'll never join you!" Just like Luke did. And then I could have thrown myself out his window rather than accept his outstretched hand.

Dr. Organ must have known what General Surgery had going against it. If the rumors about Ears, Nose, and Tennis (ENT) were true, leaving G-surge wouldn't cause any regret. Home call. Few emergencies. Decent hours. It sounded a little like living.

*

Night call brought me back to the harsh reality of G-surge.

I started in the recovery room with Ms. York. Dr. Fagan had just finished rerouting some arteries in her leg. She saddened me; she was moving the opposite direction of the recovering alcoholic with gallstones. She was only in her forties, but already suffering the late stage effects of diabetes: vascular disease, kidney impairment, and retinal damage. She had a long history of noncompliance, and even as she was losing her vision she refused to properly monitor her sugars and take her meds. She didn't even pull her long black hair away from her face. Her lack of self-respect bewildered me. However, when it came down to a choice between creating a new blood supply to her left foot or having it cut off, she consented to arterial bypass surgery.

Her blood pressure was low, so I gave her a fluid bolus. The low blood pressure surprised me; she almost always had high pressure since her blood-pressure meds were one of the pills she wouldn't take. Once the fluid was in, her blood pressure returned to normal.

The EKG chime made me look up. Ms. York's heart rate had jumped up, but went immediately back to normal.

If I hadn't been there, no one would have seen it. I examined the jagged green lines crossing the screen, the same jagged lines accompanying the beeps in the opening credits of every hospital-based TV show since beginning of time. Her green lines looked normal.

She was still groggy from the anesthesia. I didn't want to disturb her, as she was tucked up to her chin in warm blankets. "Ms. York, how are you feeling?"

"Fine." She didn't open her eyes. She adjusted her position and fell back asleep.

Everyone is fine...She might have just had a heart attack, but she's fine. I didn't trust her or the machine. I immediately sent for an official EKG and some stat labs.

When the blood vessels to your foot are in such lousy shape that your toes are gangrenous, chances are your coronaries suck too. Her bypass surgery established blood flow from her knee down to her foot, but maybe her heart needed a bypass, too.

Her new EKG looked normal, but I ordered the labs anyway. The tests were sensitive to detecting cardiac damages, and I wanted to make sure her electrolytes were normal. It is poor form to have your patient survive surgery and then die in the recovery room.

I watched her a few more minutes. Her pressure stayed up, her heart rate was normal, and she had no complaints, so I left her to go do Sleep Rounds on other patients.

No, I didn't go around waking up patients. I made sure they were tucked in so I could get some sleep. Otherwise, the nurses would wake me throughout the night asking if Mr. So-and-So could have something to help him sleep, or if Mrs. What's-Her-Name could have something stronger for pain.

I checked for Ms. York's labs twice during the next ninety minutes. The notoriously slow lab lived up to its reputation. Then I got a call from the floor nurse. Ms. York had another episode of low blood pressure. I went to her room.

She was fine. Well, not perfect. But she was more awake. She still hadn't bothered to brush her hair away from her dark eyes. She had the same monotonous, apathetic voice as before the surgery. This was the same Ms. York I had briefly met a few days earlier in clinic.

A doctor once told me, "If you look at a patient and feel depressed, then that patient is depressed."

"You seem depressed, Ms. York."

"I don't want to be alive." She delivered the statement without expression. With her pale skin it appeared that she was wearing a mask—I didn't see any facial muscles move when she said it.

"What's going on? This operation isn't the end of your life." She obviously didn't know Dr. Roland's thoughts on making such a statement. Self-condemnation is a no-no.

Nothing. She didn't even look at me. She had damaged vision from her diabetes but that wouldn't prevent her from directing her gaze my way.

She denied feeling suicidal.

"Would you like to talk to a psychiatrist? He could probably help you."

"That would be fine. Can I drink water?"

That would be fine. I suspected she said it just to placate me. I went to get her a cup of water and a psych consult. Something didn't seem right. Maybe the shrink would have better luck than I, but at the same time my gut said she suffered more than depression. But my gut wasn't giving out diagnoses.

I went downstairs to "load the boat." I found Franklin. He suggested that I run the full gamut of labs to make sure I wasn't missing anything. I told him the results were already pending. His input was worthless, but at least I wasn't going to sink alone.

I started back upstairs when the alarm sounded.

"Code Blue, TCU," a woman announced over the P.A.

"I hope this isn't her," I said to Franklin. He smiled. I hated that smile. It's usually the last thing you saw before he disappeared, like the Cheshire Cat. I turned and ran upstairs; no pit stops, no elevators.

It was Ms. York.

I entered the room as an anesthetist prepared to intubate her. A slender nurse leaned over Ms. York, putting all her weight into delivering chest compressions. Someone started another IV. People ran around putting whatever they had in their hands into the right place. Someone else stripped the sheets off the lower half of the bed.

I noticed the pulse oximeter wasn't picking up a heart rate or the oxygen saturation. I repositioned it, asking, "What happened?"

"I came in the room and she was like this." The nurse frantically circled the room. I wondered if it was her first real code.

"Not breathing and no heart rate?"

205

"Yes."

Impossible. I just talked to her ten minutes ago.

"Who is the MD running this code?" the anesthetist called out. She looked in my direction.

I glanced over my shoulder. Crap. I was the only MD in the room. The Code Blue response team hadn't arrived yet? Where were they? Where had Franklin gone, and why hadn't he followed me up here?

"I am," I said, and shivered. I felt like the team mascot sent up to bat. Wait, everyone, I'm the intern! This is a mistake; don't you care?

"We're just about to give the first Epi," the anesthetist informed me. Epinephrine revs up the heart.

"Do we know her heart isn't beating?" I asked the nurse giving chest compressions.

"It doesn't matter, Epi can't hurt her," the anesthetist answered.

"She's pulseless," said the nurse between thrusts.

"Give the Epi. Get the EKG leads on," I ordered. Someone retrieved the paddles off the crash cart that held the defibrillator. The mnemonic popped into my head: White right, Smoke over Fire. The leads went on: the white one to the right arm, black (smoke) to the left arm, and the red (fire) to the left chest. A nurse slapped two orange pads onto her bare chest. I noticed she had a few dark hairs at the edge of her nipples.

"Giving the first Epi," someone called out. Everything had to be called out so the recorder could write it down. I stood at the head of the bed next to the anesthetist. She fiddled with the endotracheal tube. The respiratory therapist, the quiet, bald guy I freaked out when I bumped the bed during the brain death exam, stood attentively next to the patient, bagging her after every fifth chest compression. The nurse on his side vigorously compressed Ms. York's chest. A third nurse at the foot of the bed was the one who wrote everything down. Another nurse readied medications on a cart off to the side. And a handful of people lined the wall, acting like they were waiting to help, but probably just watching out of morbid curiosity. We were crowded; funny how people don't get claustrophobic if they are sufficiently entertained.

I ordered the nurse to stop giving compressions. I needed to verify that her heart had stopped.

Everyone looked at the monitor, waiting for the rhythm to appear.

No one blinked; we all wanted to see it first. Everyone silently prayed it would be normal. Then we could all be doing anything but this. Why was I the one on call?

The little green line zigzagged across the black screen. The rhythm was v-fib, or ventricular fibrillation, according to the medical textbook. She needed to be shocked. I recalled the mnemonic for this, too. Shock, Shock, Shock, Everybody Shock, Little Shock, Big Shock…or something like that. They change it every year.

Before I could say anything, half a dozen people called out, "Shock!"

"Clear the bed," yelled the nurse putting the paddles on the orange pads. Everyone took a step away. For a second, the respiratory therapist stopped bagging her. No one touched the bed.

"Okay, clear. One, two, three, shock," he said. Her body jolted and immediately slumped back into its resting state. But the rhythm didn't change. V-fib can't pump blood. V-fib is the heart shivering.

The crowd thickened. This topped slowing down on the highway to look at a car accident. Here they could actually witness the miracle of death. That's where this was headed: death. When your heart stops and you stop breathing the odds are overwhelmingly in your favor that you will die. I wanted more than anything at that moment to be the hero, to lay my hands on her and have her wake up. To make her the one in a hundred that lives. She'd thank me. She'd tell me she had a newfound respect for life, a newfound respect for herself. But my gut knew that wasn't true, and I knew to trust my gut. The TV shows lie; the patient won't wake up after the hero thumps her on the chest. When you see your favorite actor push a few times on the victim's chest and give him a breath, that's not even CPR. To make a heart "beat" you need to push hard enough to compress it through the rib cage. If you don't break a rib while compressing, you probably aren't giving adequate compressions. That's why I hate compressing. The sound and the feel of breaking bones gives me the willies.

I pointed at a nurse watching from the hallway. "Go call Dr. Reed right now and tell him to get up here." I needed someone more senior than me. I wasn't on Dr. Reed's service, but I remembered seeing him the hallway an hour earlier. He could come captain this sinking ship. Load the boat! Never go down alone! Why was I still the only doctor here? We could keep pretending she was alive until he got here.

"Getting ready to shock again, everyone clear!" the nurse called.

Shock. Her body lurched.

No change.

Come on. I'll be your best friend if your heart beats.

"Another shock," he called out.

One of the nurses at the end of the bed had her hand resting on the footboard. "Get your hand off the bed," I barked. Electrocuting nurses is poor form, too.

A bunch of glares shot her way.

"Okay, clear."

Another shock. No good. I'd rather do fifty rectal exams than be here.

I noticed an ER intern at the door, looking at a note card. Then Franklin walked in. I expected him to take over—he was my senior, after all—but he just stood next to me. ARRGH! Evan's words popped into my head. Intern of the Year? My ass. I supposed he would call out any ideas. I was following the protocol anyway. The crash cart came with a laminated instruction card for codes. That way untrained monkeys, such as myself, could still follow the algorithm.

"Time for the second Epi."

"Let me get this tube in," the anesthetist said. She put the endotracheal tube down. A little bit of frothy spit appeared in it as the chest compressions continued. When they gave her the first bagged respiration, a gush of watery fluid came back. It was in the esophagus. Couldn't anything go right?

Three people listened to the chest and abdomen as the RT gave her a breath. "You're in the stomach," one of the nurses said.

"It looked like I was in the trachea," the anesthetist defended. "Maybe she has pulmonary edema. Let me listen."

Stop being an idiot. Maybe she has pulmonary edema? Can't you see, no, smell the gastric juice coming out of it? Christ, we didn't have time for this.

But I didn't say anything. It was my duty to be the calmest person in the room. The anesthetist would discover her folly in just a second. I could wait. The patient wasn't complaining either.

She listened. "I just don't know. That means I have to do it again.

If you don't know, redo it."

About time.

She put the tube in the right hole. We kept doing chest compressions, administering drugs, and giving shocks to no avail. In a previous trauma case, I had been digging through the bowels, looking for the source of bleeding in a woman who had shot herself in the stomach in a suicide attempt. The trauma surgeon looked across the table at me and asked if this was exciting. "Yeah," I had answered. What's not exciting about mucking through the bowels looking for bullet holes?

He said, "This doesn't excite me, it scares me."

Now I know what he meant. It was exciting to watch, and exciting to help, but it wasn't exciting to be the one responsible. Dying people weren't fun; they were scary.

Brad Reed, the trauma chief, showed up. His head was a bald beacon cutting through onlookers: Help is on the way! I filled him in on the situation and he took over. He called for some more drugs and shocks, but the patient went into asystole, which means no electrical activity in the heart. We tried even more drugs.

I felt progressively sicker to my stomach. It was like that feeling you get the first time you scratch your parents' car, multiplied by a million.

Reed called the code. No one disagreed. The EKG flatlined.

The recorder called out, "33 minutes," meaning we just tried to save her life for 33 minutes before calling the fight in favor of the Reaper.

That hadn't felt like 33 minutes.

The RT stopped bagging. The nurse stopped compressing. Someone turned the defibrillator off. Long faces shuffled out of the room quietly. We were the losing team.

I couldn't believe it. I had just seen her alive.

Two nurses stayed behind to clean up the mess. The crash cart needed to be immediately restocked and reorganized, as there was no telling how soon it would be needed again.

Brad pulled me aside in the hallway. He looked only a few years my senior, but it felt like I was talking to someone much older. Every time I saw him he was mulling over something serious. I never want to look like that, but events like these probably aged a person. Brad also had that ring of hair from one ear around the back to the other ear; my grandpa had that. I hope that didn't happen to me either.

I told him everything we did.

"This is the type of thing you'll get sued over," he responded. There wasn't any hint of an ill-timed bad joke in his eyes, nor did we know each other well enough to joke around at a time like this.

"Great." Thanks for adding to my misery.

"They sue everyone whose name is on the chart. I am still involved with a case from when I was an intern four years ago."

Why was he telling me this? Why was I going to get sued? I had done what I could.

Franklin looked upset, too. But no one comforted us. We weren't patients and we weren't family. We didn't count.

We sat somberly at the nurse's station filling out paperwork while Brad called Dr. Fagan, Ms. York's attending physician. After he hung up the phone he told me, "Don't brood. It is unbecoming of you. You are a good intern. Things like this happen. You just have to go on. I'll call the coroner for you." He got up and left.

That was it; no pow-wow to discuss what had happened. When a classmate died in my high school, they canceled classes, they had guidance counselors available, and other teachers offered their time to talk with any student that wanted. Now that I was in a subculture that didn't bat an eye at death; I didn't have to deal with those things. Instead, in a couple of hours I'd be teased, "That's one way to get patients off your service."

Thanks.

Whenever someone died within 24 hours of an operation, it became a coroner's case; he had to figure out what had happened. Ms. York's family didn't have long before her body would be taken to the county morgue. Just like that, she had gone from person to body. She had changed pronoun status: from "she" to "it."

I waited for her family members to show up. The operating surgeon, Dr. Fagan, didn't bother coming in to talk to them. I was the only one who had met any of them before, so Brad and Franklin disappeared. Why they allowed a twenty-five year old kid to be the medical representative, I have no idea.

I waited around the nurse's station for the family to arrive. I peeked my head in the room only once. The nurse had cleaned it, leaving the empty, sterile appearance you would expect in a hospital room. Ms. York was tucked in bed under the white covers, not unlike how she was just after surgery. Except now she had the endotracheal tube sticking out of her mouth. It is illegal to alter the body before the coroner does his exam. No matter how odd or disturbing it must be for the family to see a piece of plastic tubing protruding from their dead loved one's mouth.

Her sister, the sister's husband, and her mother arrived. The sister and the mother understood that Ms. York's life had been at risk. They had talked to Dr. Fagan before the operation. Maybe it was their interaction with him, or maybe it was how well they knew Ms. York, but they didn't appear shocked.

But the brother-in-law was more fired up. "How did this happen?" and "What happened? How could she survive the surgery but not survive a night in the hospital?" He looked like a naturally disgruntled person. At rest, his mouth turned down at the corners, a sure sign of someone who spends a lot of time frowning.

I did my best to explain what I knew. But I knew very little. The answers to his questions depended on the coroner's findings.

"Does she have to have an autopsy?" he asked.

State law required anyone that died within 24 hours of surgery to undergo an autopsy.

And then I could see it in their faces. The gears were turning under the mother's gray hair and behind the sister's pretty face. Grumpy Man's eyes were piercing me. They all shared the same thought. You were the doctor here? Where's the other doctor? I'll bet someone older could have saved her. What did you do wrong? If you're a doctor, why don't you know what happened? People's hearts stop all the time on TV and they do fine.

I wanted to say that I was sorry. But, coupled with the fact that I couldn't tell them what exactly happened, I thought it would sound like an apology rather than sympathy. Saying sorry sounded more like saying "sue me."

And then I wanted to tell them her last words. Not the glass of water part, the "I don't want to be alive" part. Then they would stop looking at me like I was a blundering idiot. But I couldn't convince myself that the family would be happy to hear that she got what she wanted. Instead I left it as a probable heart attack.

I couldn't sleep that night. And it was more than the crinkly, plastic mattress on the call room bed. Dr. Roland's soundbite about every patient that said he was going to die did. Ms. York said it, in a way.

I kept replaying the event. I didn't like being the last person to see her alive. There is a heaviness that comes with that. I knew her last words. I had the last image of her alive in my brain and now I would have to carry it forever.

During my second year of medical school, a doctor spoke to us about something or another; the one thing I remembered was his opening statement. "During the course of your practice you will kill someone. You will be extremely lucky if it is only one person."

Was this my fault? I didn't know how I would deal with that. Had I killed her? This must be what the lecturer meant; you weren't going to kill someone by "slipping" with the knife and accidentally cutting out their heart; you were going to kill someone by missing something subtle. Something that was there and you just didn't do the right thing in time.

If only I hadn't been on call that night. If only I hadn't been on that rotation. I had a million "if only" thoughts. There were so many possible ways for me to not be there. If only I hadn't been born was one of the easier ones.

I tried to focus on how I would do things differently in the future, but without the cause of death it was hard to come up with any changes. The EKG had been fine. She had been fine. Then, she was dead. There was nothing to change. And why didn't anyone say anything afterward? Was that the way to deal with this? Just shut it out? I could hear a baseball coach saying, "Son, if you dwell on the strikeouts, it will ruin your career. Think about the home runs. It's the homers the crowd wants to see; that's what they'll remember."

But, Coach, you'd be happy if I hit .350. I'm supposed to bat a thousand. Every patient that walked through the door wanted me to hit a homer. There was a league of lawyers just waiting for me to strike out. It disturbed me to think that I tried to save someone's life and someone would want me to pay for it. Of course I was going to dwell on it. What went wrong?

The next morning, at the end of rounds, Dr. Organ stopped as he was walking past Franklin and me. I thought he had something to say about last night's death, but instead he was still thinking about me being a general surgeon. "This is your chance to change him," he said to

Franklin.

Franklin shrugged and said something about bringing a horse to water.

Dr. Organ turned to me, "Are you sure you want to be a nose picker the rest of your life?"

"Dr. Organ, if we are going to call surgeons names by the orifice they probe most often, I don't think general surgeons will have the last laugh."

He looked at me and then grinned. "Okay, okay." He shook his head as he walked away.

Boy, was I ever the grinning fool. Zing! Can you feel that, buddy? But the victory was short-lived. Why was he teasing me about my future profession instead of asking me about last night?

The whole day I walked around waiting for the other shoe to drop. None of the attendings called me to their office to talk about what had happened. Dr. Fagan disregarded me just like any other day.

But no answer came. No one said anything.

Did I kill that woman?

Rachel was a sympathetic ear. Despite her biased position, I wanted to believe her that I had done everything right. At least she didn't tease me.

Chapter 43

Later that morning I ended up with Dr. Fagan in a case nearly identical to the one he did on Ms. York. Nothing was different from the day before when I assisted on Ms. York's case. As usual, I didn't exist.

"All these arteries are shit," he complained.

I was stuck watching Dr. Fagan dig around some guy's leg looking for a healthy artery when I made an amazing discovery. Well, it is a discovery in the way Columbus "discovered" America. It was always there. I discovered "stealing = genitals." Go ahead, rearrange the letters. It works.

Everyone is born with a gift. Some people can high jump, others play the oboe, and I manipulate letters, numbers, and shapes. It comes naturally. Words that look like normal words hide secrets. Look at "general." See it? It's "enlarge."

It's too bad computers have replaced ("parceled") savants. Years ago people got a kick out of odd mental ("lament") feats. No one is impressed anymore if a guy can multiply 864 by 7112 in his head. Any kid can reach into his backpack and pull out a calculator to do that.

"Are you even watching what I'm doing? Retract over here." Fagan whined.

Now, what was I thinking? Something, what was it?

Vascular surgery sucks.

Dr. Fagan spent another hour trying to find a distal artery that he could anastomose (sew together) the bypass graft to. I wished I had the power to heal. It wouldn't have to involve glowing golden light emanating from where my hands touched the body, though it'd be a lot cooler if it did. I could just touch the patient's body and have the vessels grow back as healthy as they were twenty years before. But I wouldn't want to just heal people; I want to be able to see the problem inside and watch it reverse itself.

Pretty soon the whole world would be knocking at my door to heal them. Would I have to discriminate who I healed? Who would I be to judge the good from the bad? Would some lunatic want to kill me because I threatened his personal beliefs?

But I would take those problems if I could just end this futile case. I watched Dr. Fagan piddle with the wimpy vessels. Of course, if I were to have the power to help him today, then I better have had it yesterday

214

too.

Dr. Fagan, did I kill that woman?

No, you were doing everything you could. She just had bad protoplasm. Her vessels were shit.

Thanks, that makes me feel better.

*

After the case, Brad flagged me down in the hallway. I expected him to give me the name of a good lawyer.

"Did you talk to Dr. Fagan about that code the other night?"

"No, no one's said anything. I've been waiting in limbo."

"Well, he and some of the other attendings looked over the chart and they think it looks like she died from a massive MI." A myocardial infarction was the physician's exclusionary way of referring to a heart attack so nobody knew what he or she was talking about. "They thought you did everything right."

I sighed as the stone was lifted off my chest. I could breathe again. Fagan could have said something, anything, during the case.

"Were you involved with this morning's death?" Brad asked.

I shook my head no. I wasn't even aware another patient had died.

"That's good. I thought if you were I would have to get you a skull and crossbones patch for your shoulder."

That was it. Dr. Fagan never said anything to me: no questions and no explanations. That was the worst part about medicine. You never got the answer key to correct your mistakes. What was the point of making mistakes if you couldn't learn from them?

When I called the coroner's office, the secretary couldn't find the report. She told me to call back another day.

Chapter 44

My mom finally heard from my sister. She had rented an apartment and started working full-time at a record store. My mom said it sounded like she was doing well, but the conversation eventually came to its usual point: She needed money.

Psychiatry interested me, but it frustrated me. I constantly asked, "Why can't they see what's wrong?" I was too logical to try to comprehend the power of addiction. I was too naive to understand what it is like to be held captive by an alien thought.

But I did understand one thing. Hope, not threat, was the most powerful motivator in the world. If people knew the threat, they would only hope to avoid the consequences. Wasn't that how criminals thought? Wasn't that how smokers thought? They knew the threat but hoped for the best. Logic did not move people, but hope got people to cross oceans or get off the couch to buy lottery tickets.

I really hoped my sister decided to stay clean.

Chapter 45

It was day 183. 183 times 2 is 366. I just passed the halfway point.

The clock does not stop!

Halfway through the year and I hardly knew the people in my program. It was as if we were all adventurers exploring a new planet. Occasionally our paths crossed and we shared exciting stories, but nothing personal. At the same time, we had to trust one another every night. People I'd never shared a laugh with signed out to me on a regular basis. People whose middle names I didn't know were taking care of my patients overnight. Did the Pony Express messengers ever get to know one another?

I did not know anyone on a personal level except Corey. He didn't overcome his fear of refried beans until he was twenty. When he was little, his older brother had told him that the way they made them was to feed normal beans to cows...

He seemed right about finding solace in a good relationship. Rachel became my crutch, my psychologist, and my cheerleader. My phone bill singularly accounted for half of AT&T's quarterly profits. Chatting and joking with her on the phone relaxed me, so it was worth the cost.

She nicknamed me Salsa, which gave me a welcomed escape from my doctor identity. When she called me Salsa I was no longer an overworked intern; I was a happy boyfriend who tasted great with tortilla chips.

Rachel started looking into Masters of Public Health programs in the Bay Area. There were a few in San Francisco, and Berkeley had one. She preferred Berkeley because of their reputation. Her ultimate plan was to work at the CDC, solving outbreaks. I didn't know if the CDC had branches, or it meant that it would be my turn to move, to Atlanta, some day in the future.

Chapter 46

I somehow missed the Christmas season. Oh, wait, I know how I missed it. I stayed trapped inside the hospital. Its dreary walls protected its denizens from Christmas joy. As a busy intern I easily dodged the barrage of holiday advertisements by skirting from patient to patient. Furthermore, I didn't succumb to the Yuletide materialism, as I had neither the time nor money to indulge in "must have" items required to maintain social status. Finally, patients stuck in the hospital didn't exactly emit holiday cheer.

Despite being a certified Grinch (I have always said if Christmas music was good, we'd listen to it all year round), I appreciated the importance of being with family. Back in Wisconsin a slew of relatives gathered for Christmas Eve while I sat in the call room. I missed out on my great aunt's homemade lasagna—arguably the best in the world. Instead, I got to admit other poor souls that would find themselves stuck in the hospital for Christmas.

I took Megacall that day. I covered the inpatient General Surgery patients and the Urology/Neurosurgery/Otolaryngology admissions, inpatients, and consults. Covering that many patients guaranteed I wouldn't get any rest, but the trade-off was worth it. I only had six call days the whole month.

The hospital stayed quiet on big holidays. Nobody wanted to waste time off work going to the hospital. But, it also meant that the people who did come in were really sick. All of the slightly ill people would wait until the day after Christmas to come in.

I received my first consult at 7 p.m. The trauma service couldn't get a Foley catheter into a patient. That sort of consult seemed to be a joke. If they couldn't pass a tube into someone's bladder, what made them think I could? The next option was a suprapubic catheter and they knew how to put one in. (Straight through the skin under the belly button and into the bladder.)

But the consultation protected their butts. They could do it, but if something went wrong, the lawyers would have a field day because they weren't urologists. The result? The trauma team wasted the urologist's time. Even if the "urologist" was an intern, not actually board certified in anything.

The man couldn't pee for two reasons. The first was his HUGE prostate gland. I believe the prostate gland is an argument against the existence of God as the Creator. A little common sense says don't run the pee tube through a gland that can swell up and occlude it.

(Reminds me of a joke: Three engineers were debating God's postgraduate education. One said, "God is clearly a mechanical engineer. Just look at how the muscles and skeleton work. The entire body is a brilliant system of levers."

"No, no, no," the second one said. "God must be an electrical engineer. Look at the nervous system and how intricate it is. Motor output is constantly regulated by the sensory input in a highly efficient manner."

The third one disagreed. "God is clearly a civil engineer. Who else would run a sewage system through a recreational area?")

The second reason the man couldn't pee was because he had a neurologic injury. He immediately became my neurosurgery consult. Two for the price of one.

Mr. Warner was an eighty-one year old man walking to his house when he suddenly fell forward. He probably passed out first, because when he fell he didn't brace his fall and smashed his face into the pavement. Conscious people tend to protect themselves. The paramedics found him unresponsive. They intubated him on the way in.

As the trauma team began their work-up they discovered his enlarged prostate, which got me into the loop. As they continued their work-up, they didn't find any evidence of a stroke or intracranial bleeding. The team transferred Mr. Warner, still unresponsive, to the ICU.

He looked like a corpse sucking on a garden hose. He was intubated and lying absolutely flat on the bed. Usually the head of the bed is up, a more natural position that facilitates conversation. I walked up to his face. Gaudy purple bruises underlined his eyes and the bridge of his nose had a scrape across it. A cervical collar held his neck in place. Too bad he was so scrawny; fat would have cushioned his fall. Of course, fat people don't live to eighty-one.

"Hello, Mr. Warner."

He opened his eyes. So much for being unresponsive. That seemed to happen a lot.

I asked if he could understand me and he nodded his eyes yes.

"I'm Dr. Iaquinta. I am on the neurosurgery service. The

neurosurgeon and I will look over all the films they have taken and try to figure out what is wrong. But first a couple of questions and a brief exam."

Another eye nod.

"Can you move your body?"

His eyes went side to side: No.

"Can you feel anything?" I asked.

No.

"Are you comfortable right now? Is the pain controlled?"

Yes.

I grabbed his right hand and his arm came up off the bed like a ragdoll's. I pinched his fingertips. He didn't wince. I uncovered his feet and brushed the bottom of his foot. I searched him for normal reflexes. None. He had no tone below his neck.

Spinal shock. His exam and the fact that he couldn't breathe suggested he had damaged his spinal cord in the upper neck.

"I am going to go look at those films and figure out what is going on."

Yes.

I gathered up the films and called Dr. Blanchard.

Mr. Warner was screwed. I had spent the last two days complaining about being overworked and missing out on lasagna and here was a guy trapped in his body. Where was my perspective? My mom had taught me perspective. If I cut my finger and complained, she'd say, "Oh my! Your finger is going to fall off, probably your entire hand. Oh well, I hope you enjoyed it while you had it."

"No, mom, it's just a little cut." So, my mood has suffered a little cut, but this guy was going to die.

"At least he's eighty-one," Dr. Blanchard muttered as he held up the film.

Mr. Warner had broken his second vertebra. The spinal cord had been severely and irreversibly damaged.

Dr. Blanchard and I explained to the family what had happened. They went into shock. Telling a family that their dad was paralyzed from falling over wasn't something people could take in quickly. Dr.

Blanchard continued to explain what needed to be done, but I'm sure they didn't hear it.

We gathered up cervical immobilization supplies and went to talk to Mr. Warner. Blanchard explained to him that he would be paralyzed from the neck down for the rest of his life. He would need a tracheotomy. He would need a ventilator. He would probably get pneumonia. Dr. Blanchard didn't add that he'd probably die from pneumonia.

Mr. Warner began to cry. He couldn't even wipe or shake the tears away from his eyes. He was lying so flat that they puddled next to his nose. I grabbed a tissue and blotted gently.

The head immobilizer had to be screwed into the skull. I felt guilty hurting the only part of his body that still had sensation. Some Christmas Eve.

While I attached the metal lattice to the head of the bed, Brad, the trauma chief, came in. He started laughing.

"What are these?" He jabbed me in the waist. I could tell my boxers were showing.

"They're boxers."

"Pink elephant boxers? You are one weird guy."

"What are you talking about? Pink elephants are cool." That statement would go down in the records as an argument against my heterosexuality.

Both Brad and Dr. Blanchard started laughing.

While the man in the bed next to us sat frightened to death about being paralyzed, they laughed about my choice of undergarment. I tried bulging my eyes at Brad to make him stop. I nodded in Mr. Warner's direction. I sped up tightening the brace; I had to get them out of there.

As we walked away from the room Dr. Blanchard said, "It's too bad the paramedics got there so quickly."

I'd have rather suffocated, too. Now he'd have to wait until he got a fatal infection, trapped in a motionless body.

Rotten Christmas Eve. I made two Christmas wishes. The first: If that ever happened to me, I hoped I would die before help arrived. The second: I hoped I never got so jaded or numb that I could joke around in front of a patient who is scared out of his mind.

221

INTERMISSION 2: VACATION

Chapter 47

January was my month of vacation. Rachel and I were lucky; she was off for part of the month before the next semester of med school started.

The two of us went snowboarding at Whistler. She was a former snowboard instructor and I was a newbie. After an hour of teaching, which she spent observing me fall repeatedly, she stated, "I think it would be healthier for our relationship if I left you alone for a while."

A few more hours later and I was a pro, but that didn't stop me from milking every bit of massage I could get out of Rachel that evening. You know what it leads to...

After Whistler, I spent most of my time in Madison at her place. I didn't miss the hospital one bit. In fact, I didn't want to go back. But, despite the welcome break, I had no doubts that I still wanted to be a surgeon. Deep down there was a growing satisfaction of being able to fix people.

I considered the year an anomaly. In six months I'd switch into an otolaryngology program. It couldn't be anything like internship.

Right?

I took the time to catch up with some medical school classmates. They all had horrible stories. One classmate had given a patient a weekend pass from the psych ward and the patient had committed suicide. Another had been asked to take a leave of absence from her program. She had been depressed and started making mistakes that caught everyone else's attention. The autonomy scared her; she didn't like the responsibility. She couldn't make decisions. And she hated treating people like animals; she wanted to be their friend.

Another friend waited for his Match results. The Match allocates medical students to residency programs. He hadn't matched into Urology, which was what he wanted, so he had taken a transitional surgery spot for the year so he could reapply. A transitional surgery spot is a one-year obligation to be the warm body everyone bosses around. I was in a transitional surgery spot, but I had a place reserved in an ENT program.

The Match replaced interviewing and waiting for job offers. It used to be that one program director would call another and say he had someone that would like to interview there. My impression was that everything had been done over golf or under-the-table transactions, at least for the esteemed positions. That wasn't fair, so they had set-up the Match. It concealed everything nicely.

To get an ENT spot, I had filled out a universal application and sent it to a central application service that charged me a ridiculous sum of money to forward it to the programs I selected. The average person applies to 36 programs (out of 103). A few specialties didn't have the central application, which required extra hours to fill out numerous applications. Most other specialties were not as competitive, so fewer applications were required. ENT had 243 available positions nationwide my year. General surgery had roughly 1200 and family practice had about a million.

Every program received about ninety similar applications. Then they offered 25 interviews for two positions. This varied, of course; some programs had one spot and granted 12 interviews and others did 40 for three spots. An interview offer could be facilitated by your program director calling the director of another program to "move things along," which was the very thing the Match was supposed to avoid.

I didn't get help, but I still got interviews. I went to thirteen of them scattered across the country. I scheduled and paid for everything myself in between completing my fourth year rotations.

The actual interviews should have triggered extreme nervousness, but after the first interview, I caught on. Doctors were not interviewers; they were doctors. They were used to the goal-directed questioning required to discover a diagnosis. They stumbled to make up questions in the open-ended interview. So, they created a master list, ask the same questions to every interviewee, and scored them on some bogus rating system. Many created an objective scoring system because they weren't trained to process subjective information.

I learned quickly to take control of the interviews. I got them to talk about themselves. Then, they didn't "pimp" me. I distracted them from asking me difficult questions about a field I hadn't studied yet. Anyone engrossed in telling me about his last vacation didn't notice my nervousness or that I flunked half my classes. That's a joke; two-thirds.

The one thing that separated my application from the rest was the space under Extracurricular Activities. I crammed it full. Painting, sculpting, jewelry making, drawing a comic strip, carpentry, puzzles, basketball, and ultimate Frisbee. In my breast pocket I carried photographs of things I had made, and whenever I could, I changed to subject to that photo collection.

I remember a few interview highlights. One program had the applicants carve a bar of soap with a scalpel. We were all given pictures of an object and told to "go at it."

(WARNING: When someone says, "I don't mean to toot my own horn," that means they are going to blow it as loudly as possible.)

I don't mean to toot my own horn, but I had the "David" of soap carvings. I had the advantage of having carved plaster as a hobby.

On a different interview, one of the directors administered some sort of psych test. He said, "Respond to what I say with the first word that comes into your mind."

"Okay," I said.

"Ted Williams."

"Baseball."

"Jesse Ventura."

"Jokester."

"The Armed Services."

"Inefficient." (Had I turned around, I would have seen a picture of him in uniform and a placard recognizing him for being the otolaryngologist to the president of the United States.)

"Religion."

"Necessary."

"Indiana."

"Dog."

"What?" He halted.

"Indiana was the dog's name. Indiana Jones got his nickname from his dog."

*

By the seventh interview, I was sick of it. Somewhere around the ninth interview a program director asked me the highly original question: "So what separates you from the other applicants?"

"I can take off my thumb." I proceeded to manipulate my fingers in that classic magic thumb fashion.

224

His eyebrows rose a little. I grinned. Fortunately, it was the last interview of the day and he had been chiseled by the eleven other applicants enough to crack a small smile.

"I also do artwork..." I reached for my pocket.

After a while the whole thing was a joke, pretty much like the rest of life.

When the whole interview process was over, I ranked the programs in order of desirability. At the same time, the residency programs ranked whom they interviewed. We both sent our lists in to the Central Application Service with a larger sum of money. Then they assigned medical students to their first ranked program if that program wanted them as one of their top picks. They worked down the lists of the students until all of the positions filled. Then, they didn't tell anyone until Match Day.

On Match Day the entire class met in a lecture hall and the dean pulled envelopes from a bag. The chosen student then went to the front of the class and opened their envelope to find out where they were going. Some people shrieked with joy and others grunted. It was a day of unbridled emotion.

I didn't do that because ENT (and Urology and Ophtho) was an "early match." I found out three months before everyone else because so many people didn't match into those fields that they had time to "scramble" into a different field. If I could go back in time, I'd have announced that I matched at the Pamela Anderson Center of Augmentative Surgery.

*

When vacation ended, I realized ordinary people only asked me the same two questions about residency. Did you really work crazy hours? The longest stretch of time I spent at the hospital was 54 hours; I did catch some sleep here and there.

The second question: Did you see people die?

At first, that surprised me. But, death separated my job from theirs. They could imagine working hard in their own way, but they couldn't imagine death as part of the job. I could see it in their eyes when I said that I'd seen people die. They thought about the last time they screwed up at work. They had been admonished, but no one had died.

Sure, it added a level of stress. What could be worse than sitting awake at night wondering if there was a way to keep Ms. York alive?

And witnessing people die made me realize my own mortality. I understood why doctors had a high suicide rate. Not only did we have stressful lives but we know our prognosis once diagnosed with a disease. Maybe suicide is better than end-stage pancreatic cancer.

My dad always thought he would die before the age fifty-five. His mom died at that age. Just fell over one day...kaput. My dad died a month before his fifty-first birthday. I always hated that he thought that way. His dad had lived until he was seventy-three. Why couldn't he have chosen that age?

I don't think it was coincidence that that was when my father died, or like Mark Twain being born and then dying when Haley's comet came around. I think he chose that death mentally. He definitely chose it that day in the hospital.

Me? A meteorite will squash me when I'm 78.

*

I unenthusiastically returned early to take the ABSITE exam (American Board of Surgery In Training Exam). One morning a year, every resident got a five-hour reprieve to take a 225-question exam. But where did they administer the test? Yes, the hospital, so we could go right back to work afterward.

The test is a big deal. Residency Programs boasted their chief's average score on their websites. The program directors needed high scores, so instead of organizing teaching sessions, they motivated the residents with threats of not renewing their yearly contract.

I found it ridiculous. Some of the smartest people in medical school went into surgery and then were pitted against one another, so that the bottom 50% lost. It didn't make much sense. Why not just make sure we all knew the essentials?

John finished the exam in two hours. The only person to finish before John was the female intern with the big muscles. She breezed through the test in 90 minutes. She was smarter than all of us; she had matched into a Family Practice residency for the next year.

Halfway through the test someone up front said, "Everyone look up here, please."

We all obeyed and a camera clicked. Behind the Nikon, Dr. Organ grinned. I'm sure he had a photo album of all those pictures and on quiet weekends he thumbed through it, reminiscing how he tortured each and every one of us.

When I was on the second-to-last question, a particularly tricky one dealing with the thyroid, I noticed someone standing beside my shoulder.

"You sure you still want to go into ENT?" Dr. Organ asked.

I didn't know if he asked because he saw me pondering a thyroid question, or just because he wanted me to stay there. "Pretty sure," I responded. No way would I give him the satisfaction of a definite answer.

PART 4: THE TRAUMA SERVICE

Chapter 48

They organized the trauma service as 24-hour shifts taken every other day. That meant I showed up by 7 a.m., took call for 24 hours, signed out, and went home the next morning at 10 a.m. (hopefully). Then I caught up on my sleep and enjoyed the afternoon before repeating the process the next morning. I lucked out; it was February, only 28 days.

I wasn't on call the first day, but I still had to come in to "get familiar with the service." We had a small service, but one of our patients was a "train wreck." The nickname was used on anyone in bad shape, but in this case he really was a train wreck. A train had hit him the week before. Mr. Beth had suffered three amputations: his whole left leg, the right leg from the thigh down, and his whole right arm. In addition, he had broken his pelvis.

I refrained from asking anyone how the accident happened. But then I bumped into the wound care nurse at the local video store. She held a fresh cup of coffee from the neighboring coffee shop. Coffee in the afternoon, no wonder she was always so energetic.

I found her oddly attractive despite the fact that she was probably twenty years my senior. She had blonde hair and full lips, but it wasn't her looks. I liked the way she talked. She wasn't afraid to call it what it was. Whatever it was.

"There are a lot of horrible wounds in the hospital right now."

That's what I mean. She skipped the how-bout-the-weather crap. Now that's awesome. And what a way to start a conversation on a public street!

"I know. I just started trauma service. Can you believe that guy hit by the train?"

"Isn't it terrible?"

Terrible and unbelievable. And the poor guy was a newlywed. I asked the nurse how it happened.

A noisy car went by as she replied. I convinced myself I misheard what she said.

"What?"

"He was mooning the train."

"What? Why?"

"You know, he dropped his drawers. He was standing too close to the tracks and got whacked."

"Why would someone moon the train?"

"Apparently he knew the conductor, so he was just playing a joke."

I shook my head in disbelief.

"Yeah, it's always crazy there." After a split second of reflection, she continued. "Know who else I'm seeing? The Pimp."

"The guy with the missing penis?" I whipped my head around quickly to make sure no one had heard me.

"Yes. What a pity. I took care of him a few years ago. The nurses and I used to make comments about how well endowed he was. One of the largest I ever saw." She almost had a dreamy look in her eyes. "What a shame."

"Sounds like the female race suffered a great loss." I grinned.

She smiled. "Oh well, see you later." She hopped into her black Mercedes and drove off, leaving me in a stupor.

Poor Mr. Beth. Somehow knowing his folly lessened the horror of his situation. Of course you're going to get hit by a train if you get up near the tracks and moon it. Why did knowing the circumstances of his accident lessen my sympathy when the outcome was the same?

The situations people got themselves into amazed me. And what people did to each other was worse. Didn't people know that immortality was reserved for the gods and teenagers?

The next morning's conference started out with the report of a death of a twenty-something man who was in a drugstore with a friend. The two of them had been attacked, perhaps from behind, and each was stabbed in the chest. Both were brought in by ambulance, but only one of them survived. The lucky one only had a lung punctured. The other had a hole through both his ventricles and his left lung.

The second presentation detailed the death of a 30-year-old man who was changing a flat tire when a passing car ran him over at highway speed. There wasn't much left to bring to the hospital.

The randomness scares people about death. If everyone knew they'd be squashed by very small meteorite at the age of 78 there wouldn't be any worry. People aren't scared of death; they are scared that they are going to be busy with something else when it happens. What if I die before my kids are through school? What if I die before I finish this internship, which means I spent the last year of my life working like a dog instead of traveling Italy?

Chapter 49

I spent some time with Mr. Beth, the man who had lost the battle with the train. His quick smile and light mood despite the situation convinced me he was always the life of the party. I expected him to be like Ms. York, no will to live, maybe even pleading for me to smother him when no one was looking.

The only time I heard doubt or worry in his voice was when he mentioned his wife. They married only two weeks before his accident. He confided that he hoped that it would last.

Mr. Beth asked to see his chart.

I came back with the chart and started flipping through it. "Are you looking for something in particular?"

"Is there anything about the details of the accident? I want to know where they found my limbs. How far away were they from me? What happened to them?"

Me, too.

"Here is the ER report. You were brought in with three amputations. You were confused. The paramedic said it looked like you had been dragged six blocks. Maybe it would be in a police report."

"That's a good idea, thanks."

How could a man be dragged six blocks by a train and not die?

Mr. Beth made me care about his perspective. All year I had been trying to fix people, but I rarely paused to think about more than the surgery at hand. What did the patients think? What did they worry about? How did their hospitalization change their home life? I hoped that the 22-year-old I plucked chunks of windshield out of would wear her seatbelt the rest of her life, but what else had she taken away from it? Did having her life flash before her eyes make her want to change it?

Some patients, like Hemingway, were incapable of perspective. All the trauma patients were assigned the names of famous authors as pseudonyms. This protected the victim's identity from the would-be murderers that attempted to sneak into the hospital to finish the job. No kidding.

Hemingway was unresponsive before he hit the ER door. He had fallen over backward off his barstool, out cold. No one even had to beat him up.

Patients with head and neck trauma get brought in on a stiff board and in a C-collar. The boards look like surfboards without the fins. If their pants come off easily, they are pulled off; otherwise all of their clothes are cut off.

Dr. Blanchard claimed the trauma intern had three jobs: "First, they did the rectal, then inserted the Foley catheter, and finally they pulled the arms into position for the C-spine film."

Yep, that's me. Hemingway came to just enough to try to refuse the rectal. He flexed his butt cheeks and sphincter. Trent, my chief, said with a grin, "Just stick your finger in!" Trent was a good cheerleader. He stood at the sideline watching Beetle, the new junior resident, and me run the easy cases. He looked too prim to dirty his hands on patients. His white coat was always white, a sharp contrast from his dark skin. His black hair never grew, never moved. He could have been an actor, or Alex Trebek—that guy never changes.

I cringed at the thought of a Forceful Rectal. Anywhere else they would call it sexual assault. But if we missed an injury, we would all be on the stand when the guy sobered up. A patient's family had sued one ER physician after the patient had signed out against medical advice, went home, and died. See, that's the beauty of our country; you can come to the ER for free, refuse the treatment recommended by the doctor you came to see, and then, against the doctor's advice, go home and die, and when you die, your family can sue the doctor for millions. But if you're drunk, the law says we don't have to let you go, and we get to shove our finger up your butt. In medicine we use the proverbial "we" liberally, but this rectal was all mine.

His anus was normal.

Anyway, for every "head bonk" we obtained spine films and, if they lost consciousness, a CT scan of the head, to make sure there wasn't something we couldn't see. There have been cases of people with stable neck fractures that only compress the spinal cord after the person starts moving again. This rare occurrence, coupled with the fact that most patients who come in as head traumas are too groggy, concussive, or drunk to cooperate, warranted the collars, straps, precautions, and numerous studies. And people wonder why healthcare is so expensive. There should be an ER tax on beer.

Beetle and I transported Hemingway down to the CT scanner because our time wasn't valuable enough for Highland Hospital to pay for someone else to transport patients. Yet they wouldn't give us keys to the elevator, so we had to get a nurse to come key in the floor. The administrators thought that if we had keys we would be dominating elevator usage when it was needed for patient transport. Yes, that would definitely be a problem, because I knew that if I had an elevator key to the ER elevator I would spend my free minute riding it up and down, making it difficult for patient transport to occur. Never mind that I AM THE PATIENT TRANSPORTER!

Normally, the medical student and I would do the transporting, but he disappeared around midnight. If you are ever a medical student, know this: Do not disappear when you are needed for menial tasks.

"Why don't we work more realistic shifts? This 26 hours on 22 off is killing me after one round." Only the second call and I was whining. But if I didn't whine I wouldn't have anything to say.

Beetle grunted something about there not being enough of us. Beetle looked like the mechanic who yelled out from under your car "Just a minute..." Then a loud CLANK, a muttered "Damn," and then a cheerful, "There she goes, good as new." And when he scooted out you saw his tousled hair and a grinning face that might have been shaved yesterday or the day before.

"But if you put us anywhere else on Earth, a bunch of hippie college students would be protesting that we're sweatshop labor." We really were one of the last bastions of slave labor.

"But no one in America cares. They think every doctor earns 300,000 fucking dollars. They want us to take a beating for five years as our rite to passage to riches."

Oh well, back to the important stuff. I pointed at Hemingway. "What's his BAL?" Beetle had introduced the Blood Alcohol Level guessing game on an earlier patient.

Hemingway might as well have been a corpse. He was out cold again. It amused me when drunken trauma patients received the pseudonym of an author who abused alcohol. I wonder if Ernest ever arrived to the ER passed out wearing a pair of pink fuzzy socks and what looked like the remnants of black nylons.

"Point 22," Beetle said assuredly.

"No way, point 18. You're too high. He's drunk, but he's got good teeth." Big time drinkers have nasty teeth. "He's a lightweight so he passed out earlier."

"No, the only reason his teeth are good is because he is still young. You'll see."

An hour later we played the game again with Bronte. In most states the legal limit is .08 for operating a motor vehicle. Hemingway's BAL came back .31, a point for Beetle. I guessed Bronte's BAL to be 0.22. The final answer: 0.224. My point.

If it were Prohibition, we wouldn't have anything to do except sleep.

Chapter 50

The trauma teams have a nightly ritual called Trauma Theatre. Traditionally, they watched a violent movie. Somehow, watching violence supposedly prevented it from coming in by ambulance. But I believed the opposite was true. After all, it's those violent films that make people go out and do violent things, right?

Beetle and Trent accused me of changing it to the "art film trauma theatre."

But it worked. The previous night's team had watched *Reservoir Dogs*, and that evening they had a patient die on the table as they tried to stop the bleeding from an abdominal stab wound. (During all of *Reservoir Dogs*, Tim Roth is bleeding from an abdominal wound.) We watched *Rushmore* (my non-violent choice), and our only two activations were drunk drivers. Both crashed their cars into brick walls. They don't have deer in Oakland, so people need something else to drive into in the middle of the night. Trent scored his first point in the ETOH game on the second driver.

A trauma interrupted *Twenty Dollars*. Orwell received his injuries not from the car accident he was in, but what happened right after it. He got out of his car and the person he rear-ended threw his car into reverse and purposely backed over him.

The next trauma patient had called his girlfriend and said, "I'm coming over to give you a beating. Wait there for me." While he was in transit, she called her brother, and by the time the boyfriend got there, the girl's brother and his friends beat the living daylights out of him.

People get a certain satisfaction from hearing the weird stories. It comforts them to know they aren't that messed up. That's how the nightly news works.

People doing weird things is one thing, but doing it in the middle of the night is another. I woke up to the trauma pager spitting that "a man had been found down by his neighbors with questionable loss of consciousness. ETA: four minutes."

So, after the only two hours of sleep I was going to get that night I oozed down to the trauma bay. I put on a lead vest that accounts for one-half of earth's mass and then a disposable gown and rubber gloves.

The EMTs brought the patient into the room. They tried to explain that his neighbor found him at the bottom of the stairs after hearing a thumpety-thump-thump-thud. But the patient kept yelling, "Get me out of this fucking thing. I'm fine, let me out."

The EMTs had him strapped to the body board with his head in a C-collar. We couldn't let him go. As I stated before, an inebriated person is not responsible for his health. Our country makes generous concessions regarding drunks. If a drunken person leaves a bar and runs over someone, the injured party can sue the bartender. Maybe a drug that can make you a dangerous idiot shouldn't be legal.

So there we were, obligated to care for a guy that was screaming, "Fucking mother fuckers, let me the fuck out of here." I documented it in the chart.

Beetle looked at me. "Point 33."

"Point 25." I shrugged.

We informed him that we had to take some x-rays to ensure he hadn't fractured his neck. He was too belligerent for logic. "I'm fucking fine. Look! I can move." He struggled violently in his restraints.

We waited patiently for him to stop. Wouldn't that be great if his limbs just fell flat, if he finally knocked the loose shard of bone into his spinal cord? Then I'd dance around him singing and pointing, "I told you so, I told you so."

He finally promised to lie still so we could release him from the restraints to examine his backside. We found a gash on the back of his head pouring blood into his hair. But he couldn't feel it, or the lacerations on his face. I told you, alcohol is a great anesthetic.

His blood alcohol level was 0.35. Beetle had a knack for the BAL game.

The next drunk started where the last one left off. He didn't cooperate either. In my brief experience, the more snarled your hair is, the bigger a jerk of a drunk you are. This guy was the woolly mammoth of jerks.

"Can you move your hands?" I asked.

"No."

"Move your feet," I ordered.

"I can't."

The ER attending grabbed his scissors and pinched the man's big toe between his fingers and the scissors.

"OUCH!" He kicked his foot and raised his hand. He repositioned himself on the gurney.

"Moving both feet and hands spontaneously," I called to the recorder.

"Shut up. Leave me alone, or I'll teach you a lesson." He swung at me. I dodged backward; his fist almost got my cheek.

Beetle lunged forward and grabbed his outstretched arm and in a flash had it twisted against the man's body.

"OWWWW! Let me go! Let me the fuck go!" The man whimpered. Beetle didn't let go. I could see a tear welling in the drunk's eye. I needed to learn that move.

The nurse wearing combat boots put him into restraints. She had a tattoo of a woman in combat boots on her arm. I wondered if that tattoo girl had a tattoo of a girl. Maybe she was a Norman Rockwell fan.

Our patient gave up struggling against the restraints. He turned to the poor-me routine. "C'mon, I'm not an animal. Why do you guys have me tied up like this?"

That didn't last long. As we tried to position him for his neck films he tried to insult himself free. "You are nothing, punkassmotherfucker. Look at you, scruffy man."

Beetle countered. "I'd rather be scruffy than fat."

That showed him. Ugly, you forgot ugly, Beetle. Look at his face; it's all out of proportion. Maybe he has acromegaly.

We walked behind the metal screen to protect ourselves from radiation.

"Thanks, Beetle," I said.

"Nobody beats on my intern except me."

Does the First Amendment give me permission to tell that patient he's an anus?

I know, I know. Doctors that pass judgment start thinking they're God. But, I didn't get to ground him or give him a suspension. It was more diagnosis than insult. Sir, I've figured out what's wrong with you. You are an anus.

The next patient stabbed himself in the abdomen. He feared that the Mafia was out to kill him so he figured he would be safe in the hospital. Logically. He should have given himself a vasectomy while he was at it.

All the lunacy combined with lack of sleep was affecting my feeble brain.

I discovered one of the most frightening things you can do to a slightly confused or paranoid patient. I crept into the paranoid man's room while he slept. I pulled the curtain all the way around his bed. Then, in a gravelly voice, I whispered, "Red rum." I kept repeating it, a little louder each time, until I heard him stir, then I softened my voice. When he called "Who's there?" I only answered with "Red rum." Then, I started walking around the bed pushing on the curtain with my arms.

Okay, I didn't really do that, but you can imagine.

I didn't step in to save Beetle from the next patient, a spry 97-year-old who fell at her home on the way to the bathroom. The EMTs had brought her in because there was a question of whether she had lost consciousness. She arrived at the ER awake and oriented. That's rare for a nonagenarian.

Just like the belligerent drunk guys, she started moaning about having her neck immobilized. Beetle told the woman to calm down and that he'd remove it as soon as they were certain that no damage had been done.

"When I get out of this, I am going to kick your ass," she cackled with an outstretched arm.

I was about to lunge forward and twist her arm until I realized that it was one fight I'd love to see.

I want to live long enough and be healthy enough to make threats like that.

Chapter 51

Rachel and I made up ridiculous pet names for each other. I had been calling her "fruitbean" for a while and even went so far to make up stickers with what looked like a bean-shaped apple with little green leaves on top. I stuck them onto the letters I sent her.

She decided to retaliate. The name that made me laugh the hardest was coon nut. For Valentine's Day she sent me an egg carton she had relabeled "One Dozen Grade-A Coon Nuts." Inside were walnuts with little paper raccoon heads pasted on them.

After the initial laughter subsided, I realized I couldn't have a carton of coon nuts in my house. The last thing I needed was raccoons scurrying about my already crowded one-bedroom. So, in classic alien-anthropologist fashion, I brought them to the hospital and set them in the resident's lounge to observe responses.

The first resident spotted them on the table. "Coon nuts, hmmm." He walked away.

Then, I was called away to see the best patient in the history of midnight trauma calls. I watched the EMTs transfer a skinny white kid with dreadlocks to the trauma bed. In a Jamaican accent, he said to one EMT, "Me thank you for your care, mahn."

I knew he wasn't like our other patients. He was high instead of drunk.

We cut off layers of multicolored hemp clothes. We searched through thick, matted hair for head lacerations. For a guy in a "highway speeds" car accident he'd been lucky. The EMTs made it sound like a disaster. Seeing his squashed car had sent them into a panic.

Beetle asked him, "Have you been smoking pot this evening?"

"We don't know pot; we only smoke the herb."

I laughed. He wasn't in distress; he was stoned. I asked him how a young white guy gets a Jamaican accent. He confessed he picked up his accent from his reggae friends and that he was actually from a small town up north. But, that didn't detract from his character.

"I need to do a rectal exam. It helps us determine if you have had any internal bleeding," I informed him. Actually, the position of the prostate is more important; it is rare to have a traumatic rectal injury. That is, a traumatic injury without putting something into the rectum.

"Me not going to question what you need to do, mahn."

I performed the rectal. Normal as usual.

"Me not like that, mahn."

We sent him off to x-ray. Beetle and I started writing our notes. "What was his name?" I asked.

"I never remember. If they answer I just take it as a sign that their airway is open." We gave him the nickname Rasta Man until he could supply us with a more appropriate answer.

I told him I was going to numb up his face to close his wound.

"Let me look into your eyes and see what you are made of, mahn."

Our eyes stayed locked long enough for him to peek behind the curtain.

"I'm mostly blood and guts on the inside," I kidded.

"You're selling yourself short, my friend," he said with an intense look.

I like sewing wounds closed. In minutes I take something ugly and make it pretty again, albeit with a certain Frankenstein monster look. While I sewed, Rasta man said, "Me know that you're doing beautiful work."

"How do you know that?"

"Me only sew good so me will only be reaping good."

Me sew good, too...on your face. "You believe in karma?"

"You don't believe karma, you live karma, mahn."

You live in a car? Too bad it got smashed.

The next morning after call, Beetle and I ate breakfast in the lounge. "What the hell are coon nuts? I figure it must be a regional thing. Have you ever heard of scrapple?"

"No. What's that?"

He reached across the table and grabbed a coon nut with his slender hand. "It's the stuff left over from a pig after everything else sellable is taken. It's this gelatinous gray glop that is fried. I guess some people like it. I think it's a Pennsylvania thing. Maybe coon nuts are like that."

I shrugged. It sounded worse than Corey's refried beans.

"Someone has to know what it means. Some sort of inside joke. This doesn't even look like it was bought. It looks like someone just glued some printed labels on the carton." He turned it over in his hand.

"I was thinking maybe it was some sort of bloodhound training toy. Like they smell these to know what they are supposed to go after."

I giggled.

"I saw them last night and kept having visions of raccoons burying them in the ground." He put his paws together and pretended to dig.

*

That evening I had dinner with Kendra's friend Dhara, who interned at another hospital. Some of her rotations overlapped hospitals with my rotations. We both enjoyed talking about indie movies and simply escaping the reality of the hospital.

Dhara was an attractive Indian woman and we got along well. She seemed a little depressed, but I imagined it was because she was also an intern in an Ob-Gyn (Obstetrics Gynecology) program. I made it clear to her that I had a girlfriend.

I also told Rachel about her after I had first met her. Dhara had the potential to become a real friend, instead of someone to hand off patients to at sign out. By telling Rachel everything about her, I would not only be honest, but could find out what type of girlfriend Rachel was.

When I called Rachel I got a not so subtle hint.

"How was your date with your 'other girlfriend?'" she asked.

"Ha ha. We had dinner and talked about movies. I told her all about you. She knows I have a thing for Fruitbeans."

That took the edge off the conversation but I could tell Rachel wasn't thrilled. Rachel knew a number of my good friends were women, women that I never dated, so I didn't think it was any big deal.

Chapter 52

The 2:45 a.m. page.

"Hello, Doctor, the patient you admitted from the ER needs a diagnosis on his orders."

I managed to grunt out a "Huh?"

"On his order sheet there isn't a diagnosis for us to put into the computer system."

"Fractured ribs. He broke two ribs." Time for sleep.

"I need you to write it."

What? "Why?"

"We need something to enter into the computer. We can't enter him in without a diagnosis and if we can't enter him into the computer we can't do any of his orders."

"I just told you, fractured ribs. I'll write it when I round in a few hours."

"The rules are that it has to be written."

"Well, take it as a verbal and I'll sign it when I round." I grumbled.

"No, I can't."

"Yes, you can."

"No, I can only take verbal orders for medications."

"This is foolish. This has no effect on his health care or his condition. Just take the order."

"If this were my hospital or your hospital we could do that. But this is Highland Hospital and we have to follow their rules."

"Oh, come on."

"Rules are rules."

I marched to the floor and wrote the diagnosis in large, furious letters across the top of the chart. *Rules are rules*. A sure sign of an unthinking individual.

I steamed and seethed my way back to the call room. Rules are rules! If it weren't for changing rules, you couldn't vote. How about that?

It was too late in the year for this crap. There wasn't a time or place for petty games of abuse. People like her wore out the others. People

242

like her made the good people, like Dr. Blanchard, leave. Yes, he was going to another hospital because he could no longer stand working at County.

I took a deep breath and sighed. Corey had warned me about this. And Corey also told me that no one, not even an evil nurse, could stop the clock. It was 3 a.m., the wee early hours of day 243, and the clock was still ticking forward. It just passed the two-thirds point. I could hear John Fogerty singing alternate lyrics to Proud Mary, "Big clock keep on tickin'."

Somehow the rest of the world knew the significance of that day. For the rest of the day, everyone put away the guns, drugs, knives, and alcohol. Well, almost everyone. We only had one activation and it was in the middle of the day.

I was sitting in the resident's lounge diligently reading when I heard a bang in the distance. Kendra yelled to me from her call room. "Hey, did you hear that?"

"Yeah."

"It's your next trauma patient."

"Maybe they missed."

"We'll see."

I read for the next ten minutes. The trauma pager startled me; it was obnoxiously loud. A voice cut through the static of the speaker. "Level 2 trauma. 26-year-old male GSW right thigh. Vital signs stable. ETA five minutes. Kissshht." It cut out.

Kendra called. "Told you so."

"You suck."

At some medical schools they have the third-year students put nasogastric tubes down each other just so they know what it feels like. I would have to shoot myself in order to relate to my patients. Where I grew up, if you heard a gunshot in the distance it meant it was November and someone just missed a deer.

The young, black man howled in pain. It didn't look as if he should hurt so badly. He only had a dime-sized hole in his right, lower, lateral thigh. It was hardly trickling blood. A properly placed postage stamp would conceal the wound completely.

"I'm going into shock. I'm going into shock. OhmygodamIgoingtodie?"

243

"No, you're not dying." The anesthetic effects of words are grossly overrated. The nurses couldn't start a line on him so I put one into his femoral vein.

"What are you doing? Are you putting more holes in me? Give me some pain medicine."

"We'll give you pain medicine as soon as we have an IV in you. We can't inject medicine into your blood without a line."

While I worked on the line, the x-ray tech took pictures of his leg. The nurse gave him a healthy slug of Fentanyl as soon as I got the line in. The dose she gave him would have put most people to sleep, assuming they hadn't just had their femur shattered by a bullet.

He kept writhing. "Just cut it off. Please just cut my leg off."

Trent tried to rationalize away the patient's fears. "Sir, you do not want your leg cut off. The bone doctors will fix your leg." He told the nurse, "Give him another 25 of Fentanyl."

"We already gave him 75."

"And it hasn't touched him. We'll keep giving him Fentanyl until it puts him at bay."

A few winters back there was a news story about a lone hunter whose leg had been crushed under a fallen tree. He cut off part of his leg to get free. I remember thinking the man must have just panicked and made a hasty decision. There must be a secret nerve in the leg that makes you want to cut it off when stimulated. I've got to find that nerve and name it after myself.

We unloaded him onto the orthopedic service. They didn't cut his leg off. And I returned upstairs to the lounge.

All but two of the coon nuts were gone.

*

Before we left the next morning, another GSW came in. A young woman had been shot in the head. Her heart had electrical activity, but it wasn't pumping blood. We ran the code, gave drugs, performed CPR, to no avail. A 33-year-old woman was dead.

And for the first time that month one of our murdered patients made the local news. She had recently divorced an abusive man and returned to college to finish her teaching degree. Her ex-husband hadn't let their separation stop his assaults. She placed a restraining order against him, but that hadn't stopped him either. She had complained to the police twice within the previous few weeks and her family had contacted the DA regarding the husband's persistent threats. According to the news report, the family had reported to the police that he had threatened to kill her. And that morning, after she dropped her son off at preschool, he shot her in the head as she walked from her car to her house.

Hooray justice system.

I went home depressed and called Rachel. We laughed about the coon nuts. But, then she asked, "Do you have any more plans with Dhara?"

"No, but I'm sure that we'll talk again."

"Oh." Flat answer. Silence.

I intended to be honest with Rachel. But, it was obvious she didn't approve. Rachel wouldn't say that she didn't want me to hang out with Dhara, but soon she had little jokes and jabs about my "other girlfriend." I knew it made her nervous after all; Dhara was here, Rachel was there.

"You'll like her, too." Couldn't we all just be friends?

"If you're having fantasies about a threesome, forget it."

What a wet blanket. "No, when you move out here." I tried to explain that Dhara was a cool person, not a cool potential second girlfriend.

"I've been looking into that. The counselor said this isn't the right time to do it, and by the time you came around to agreeing I had already missed the deadline for applications at Berkeley."

"Oh." Gulp.

"Yeah, I just found out, but I didn't want to say anything because you seemed depressed from having such a rough night."

I felt defeated. I immediately understood where Rachel was coming from. She knew she wasn't going to be out here for over a year. Which meant more long distance relationship and little chance of meeting Dhara. When we first met she told me she had just had a rough ending to a long distance relationship, that was supposed to translate into, so I am not going to take dating you seriously. But that didn't happen.

My expectation that Rachel would turn cartwheels because I made a new friend, a female friend, suddenly seemed as foolish as mooning a train with one foot on the tracks.

Chapter 53

Another busy weekend day. I prayed for rain, but the cursed sun wouldn't obey.

Our streak of gunshot wounds continued.

The trauma bay filled with helpers and watchers in preparation of the patient's arrival. Normally, nobody ever had time to help. But gunshot wounds were like codes; suddenly the back wall filled with spectators.

Our first patient had been shot in the butt. I expected him to be hollering more, but he screamed only when we prodded the bullet holes. That hurts. Go figure. But on trauma, the primum dictum is never ignored: Penetro totus foramen. All holes must be prodded!

The man had been shot with a magic bullet. He had escaped from a couple of muggers, but one had shot him in the left butt cheek. The bullet had entered the left side of his butt and exited the cheek near the anus. Then it entered the right cheek, turned ninety-degrees, and tracked forward through the perineum and exited just lateral to his penis. Oliver Stone could have made a movie about the path of that bullet. Second shooter!

I had to place a Foley catheter into him to evaluate for urethral trauma. For the second time that day I heard a man scream in pain as I threaded the tubing into his penis. I crunched my knees together and silently prayed I would never be conscious if I had to have one inserted. The tube passed into the bladder and clear urine returned. He didn't have a urethral injury.

This time when we went down to the CT scanner I produced an elevator key from my pocket.

"Where did you get that?" Beetle exclaimed.

I grinned like the kid that stole a cookie. "I borrowed a key from one of the nurses and ran to the local hardware store to have copies made." They couldn't hold me down.

I pulled an extra copy from my pocket and gave it to Beetle. He rewarded me with a grin even wider than my own.

The CT tech performed his job with the enthusiasm of a drill sergeant. He grabbed a rectal catheter. It was a skinny, hotdog-shaped instrument with a tube attached to it. Two-thirds the way down the hotdog was an inflatable balloon.

The tech barked to the patient, "I'm gonna stick this up your ass."

Beetle and I looked at each other and burst out laughing. Fortunately, we were far enough away and stifled ourselves enough that the patient didn't hear us. I think. I wish doctors could get away with talking like that.

The tech dangled the device in front of the patient. He inflated the balloon to a diameter of two inches. "When I do this inside your rectum you are going to feel crampy."

The patient cowered. "Man, I get shot and then I get a tube up my dick and another in my butt. This isn't my night."

Yes, the trauma didn't stop with the bullet.

When I left the hospital that morning I passed the man who had cut his drinking down to "two fifths" a day after his bout of pancreatitis. He was in a hospital gown. I feared to hear why he was admitted, so I ducked around a corner. I wanted to believe he was cutting down.

Are you reading what was going on here? The past weeks had been a constant flow of injured patients. There must be more to life than this. Don't we humans do anything besides break things and fix them and break them again?

Where was the logic in these events? People just kept getting hurt. Perhaps it was that simple. The people who didn't think got injured. I wanted a greater understanding: a rhyme, a reason. Maybe it was the patient population. The people who had good karma didn't need to go to the ER. I wasn't really helping the world. I was just patching the tires.

*

Mr. Beth, the amputee poster-boy, was the topic of discussion in social-work rounds. Every Tuesday the social workers, physical therapists, dietitians, home care coordinators, and the utilization review representative met with the interns to discuss the disposition of the patients of each surgical team, what needed to be done, and then prayed that it would happen.

His skin grafts and amputations had healed well. He needed rehabilitation. He needed to be fitted for a wheelchair; he needed to learn how to be right-handed.

If he had no other option, he would have to go to the skilled nursing facility. They could fit him for a wheelchair there and have physical therapy work with him. But the waiting list was at least three weeks long. He would have to stay here.

The bureaucratic BS didn't affect Mr. Beth's phenomenal attitude. He wanted to get out of bed. He wanted to get a wheelchair. He longed to get on with his life. Nothing could lower his spirits and nobody wanted to try. No one needed to say what we all expected to happen in the near future. If he'd been a young child, his sort of accident might have made national news, and maybe a guardian angel philanthropist would have risen from his wreckage.

I went to see him that afternoon.

"Well, the good news is that the graft has healed enough that we think you can start sitting up and even get out of bed to a wheelchair."

"Great, I'm sick of sitting here."

Mr. Beth proved there was hope for the world. If a man could lose three limbs and his wife and still wanted to get on with his life, he could do anything. Maybe the shocking thing about human nature isn't the stupid ways we hurt ourselves. We all do stupid things. Maybe the shocking thing is that we are resilient enough to try to push forward, even after suffering great failures.

If Mr. Beth was going to leave the hospital a better man, maybe I could, too.

Part 5: THE H. M. O.

Chapter 54

I left County Hospital. Forever.

I escaped that morning before the sun rose. On the way home I passed the corner where a man, a late night trauma patient, had been shot in the chest a week earlier. Six candles burnt idly on the curb.

That was the closest I had ever been to seeing a patient outside the hospital walls.

I ditched Grand Rounds (persuaded by the maxim "Physician, heal thyself") to stop by my home sweet home and sleep for two hours. A Done-with-County celebration. A "minute" for myself to double my sleep for the night. I did better than that. I fell into a coma before setting my alarm and didn't wake up until 9:30. I raced to the hospital feeling that same panic that Franklin must have felt earlier in the year.

I arrived to find the residents finishing their last conference. I got a few quizzical glances, but no one asked questions. No one cared.

Chapter 55

My new chief was Dr. Brad Reed. The last two times I had seen him had been horrible situations. He had me call Blanchard that first night of Neurosurgery call, the call that led to me sawing open a skull in the middle of the night. And he was the one who arrived at the end of Ms. York's code. The guy who said I'd probably be sued. He earned the unspoken, secret nickname The Dark Angel.

Brad had that horseshoe of short hair wrapped around his head like so many aged men. He was only 35, which isn't old, but older than most residents. He talked to the residents and attendings like they were old golfing buddies. When he wasn't chumming, he seemed falsely intense. He said to Barclay (my junior) and me, "Come here you two, we need to have a little talk." Then he put his arms out like we were going to huddle. I kept my distance; he reminded me of my dad, right before he would yell at me for leaving tools on the garage floor. Maybe it was my imaginative Italian upbringing, but the Big Boss only hugged you before he sent you to your grave.

This is what he said during our first huddle. "Let the flak fall to me. This is a system of mediocrity. Everybody is happy with the average result. Make yourselves better. Don't do things just because it is how they do it. Only a few of these attendings are great, the others just get by. Call them on what they are doing wrong. Don't give extra days of antibiotics. They do things that aren't backed by clinical evidence because of one oddball case they remember."

The attendings' tight reins bothered him; just like the other chief's he wanted to be in charge. I understood, but thought he'd be just as rigorous when he became an attending. Whenever he told me to do something, he'd say, "Don't listen to those assholes. Do it the way I said." Not exactly a sound argument, but I didn't care. I did whatever he said. Most of it was voodoo anyway, and his spells worked just as well as theirs. I figured I might as well please the person I was around the most. I was completely innocent...I only followed commands from above. Just like the Army.

Actually, there was no worry that he would be a meddlesome attending. He had made it abundantly clear that he was eager to practice privately and make "the big bucks." I wouldn't recommend going into medicine for that, but Reed would do just fine; he seemed to genuinely care about his patients as much as he cared about the money he might make.

Barclay didn't care for the group circle thing either. She only had one mood: bitter. With almost no prompting, she'd tell you why. Number one: She never threatened to quit the program, so along with Franklin, she got screwed out of good rotations. Number two: Her patients repeatedly called her nurse. Even liberal California wasn't used to seeing a young, black female doctor.

The call seemed worse than at County. By 11 a.m. I was ready to throw my pager out the window. The only people happy to hear a pager chime are the people who shouldn't have them: teenagers, drug dealers, and teenage drug dealers.

I covered a million patients that day—well, about 25, but it felt like a million. I started putting a hash mark on my census sheet for every page. Most pages were preventable if the nurse would have looked at the patient's chart before calling. Brad explained that it was the hospital's policy not to put nurses in the position of making a decision. They were supposed to follow orders and call the MD with questions.

I liked the idea of the Thinking Nurse. Why not have vigilant and knowledgeable nurses taking care of my patients? However, one of the problems with thinking is that it allows for the opportunity to misunderstand.

"Doctor, you wrote for his medicine drip to stop at ten p.m.," a woman said on the other end.

"Yes."

"Well, do you want me to stop it?"

"What was the order?" I questioned.

"Stop amiodarone drip at ten p.m."

"And what was your question?"

"Should I stop the drip?"

"What time do you have?"

"10:15."

I was positive I could keep asking questions all night without two and two meeting up to make four. But I wasn't in the mood for sick games.

"Yes, stop the drip." I started doodling fish swimming across my paper. Great, I'm turning into a madman, too.

"I don't feel comfortable stopping it."

251

"Why?"

"You just can't stop a medicine that has been on for 24 hours."

"Yes, you can."

"No, why would you just stop it?"

"Because that was his loading dose. Now we only have to give him a little every day so he maintains the same blood level. It's what cardiology recommended; read their note."

"No."

No? "Fine, but if you don't follow the order you will be responsible for what happens. If you follow the order then I am responsible. Now you do what you have to do, write me up, or whatever, but follow the order. I was just down there and I saw him. His heart rate and blood pressure are controlled. You can stop the drip."

"I don't know. I am going to call the pharmacist."

A half hour later she paged again. "The pharmacist agreed it could be stopped. Do you want me to stop it now?"

Arrg.

My four a.m. page was "Doctor, are you sleeping?"

"Yes." No, I'm sitting by the bed eagerly awaiting your page. I wouldn't dare sleep at 4 a.m.

"I wanted to let you know the Ativan is working. Mr. Trillon is resting peacefully if you wanted to change his line. But you're sleeping so you will probably want to wait a couple of hours, huh?"

"Yes." Click.

I had 62 hash marks by the time I rounded the next morning. I never watched the TV dramas, but I'm willing to bet that sort of crap never happened on ER.

There were some legitimate pages. At County we always had a few "rocks" sitting on service—patients waiting to go to a skilled nursing facility. They were easy to round on because they had no active issues. And County had drug abusers. Anyone could manage a skin abscess; just drain them and watch them heal. But the HMO patients needed to be in the hospital; they had ugly tumors, diabetes, and poor cardiac function.

After my night on call, I got to be second assistant on a 15-hour case. I discovered the exact reason why I'm going into ENT: People don't have a pancreas above the shoulders. There I was over two-thirds the way through the year and I still spent most of my time in big cases holding hooks.

There was an eighties station on. They played five U2 songs during the case. They also played two songs by "The Fixx." Neither of them was "Saved by Zero."

Brad laughed when we took off our surgical masks after the case. "We both need to shave!"

"That's what forty-hours stuck in a hospital without a razor does," I said.

"The longest I have ever gone is eleven days."

"I went six weeks once. I grew out a beard to be Obi-wan Kenobi for Halloween."

"No, I mean eleven days straight in the hospital. I've had a beard before."

"No way."

"I shit you not. I did a couple years of Neurosurgery residency before switching into this program. On one of my rotations, we would finish so late at night, so it wasn't worth it to drive back home because I only had a few hours before I needed to start rounding again."

No wonder all his hair had fallen out.

Chapter 56

"What's the difference between an intern and a puppy?"

"What?" Evan grinned.

"A puppy eventually stops whining."

That's the joke Dr. Organ's son told Evan when he worked with him. Dr. Organ's all reaching power was such that his son maintained the "Organ Presence" at the hospital where I would spend the next four years.

The fact that Dr. Organ's son was a surgeon was a surprise in itself. I expected his son would be a socially inept vagrant living halfway around the world cursing his father for such a rigorous upbringing.

Evan forewarned me about the experience. There was one rule for working with "The Organizer": Don't do anything unless he tells you. Not a single thing. He scolded me for pre-opping the patient. "Did you write the history and physical? No. So why would you want to say the patient is still ready for surgery? When you do something, think of doing it with a 'Your Honor' in front of it."

"What?"

"As in, 'Your Honor, I increased her dose of morphine.' Let me do everything; it keeps your name out of the chart. If you have any questions call me, any time of day. Do not change any orders, even if they seem trivial. No cowboy medicine, buckaroo. Just call me."

"That makes everything easy for me."

"Right."

But he didn't really want me to call him. He wanted the junior resident to call him. I already knew that another intern called him to ask permission to give one of his patients Tylenol. She never got past the point of, "You are the intern calling me?"

He spent the next half-hour grilling me on the minutiae of appendicitis. When I answered specifically he would say, "Back off Einstein, you're getting too deep. I just want the simple answers." When I gave him the simple answers, he said I wasn't specific enough. He made inferences from every statement I made, often incorrectly. He was just like his dad, always keeping the residents on their toes. But he didn't have the look of mild amusement his dad did while torturing us.

After the case, the anesthesiologist quietly commended me for "keeping my cool while working with that asshole."

But he did take the time to teach me surgical technique. Nine months into the year seemed like an appropriate time to start. He delicately handled the tissues. He scrutinized every motion I made. He used the same little sayings that his father used, except he never accused me of being from "Disney World Medical School" or giving "Mickey Mouse" answers.

I mimicked his method of sewing the layers of the wound closed before he had a chance to reiterate everything I watched him do. "This boy can learn," he said to the scrub tech. "We might get a good price for him down south."

Corey suffered a similar problem. I found him draped over a chair in the resident's office. His almost non-existent hair poked out in every direction. He was unshaven and he had a skin indentation across his forehead that proved he had worn an OR cap all day. He dragged his face upward when I entered, but didn't greet me with his usual smile and "hey man."

"What's up, Corey?"

He looked up from his chair. "I got in big trouble today."

"You got yelled at for not shaving while on call?"

"I never even had the time. I've been so busy. And I think I am going to get fired again."

His voice shook. His right leg shook faster than his voice. I had never seen Corey scared.

An attending kicked Corey out of the OR during a frustrating case.

"All I was doing was retracting. That's all I ever do in there. The dissection wasn't going his way. Next, he yelled at me to quit being so passive aggressive. Then, he stood up and shouted in my face, 'FUCK YOU!'"

Of course Corey would clash with Dr. Landa. Dr. Landa had recently proclaimed himself "the prince of 3 a.m. surgery." With Corey's giant forehead, he couldn't work next to a surgeon with such a big head.

Corey continued, "I said, 'Sir, the patient needs you to finish this case. '" I could see it perfectly. Corey knew not to argue, but would still think he had won with that comment. Dr. Landa refused to work with him and kicked him out of the OR.

"In the past few weeks I've watched that guy cut the phrenic nerve, cut the pulmonary artery twice, and transect the bladder. I know I'll take the blame at M&M. But, anyone in that room knows that I stand there for hours like this." He leaned away from the invisible table and stretched one arm toward it, just as I do when I'm retracting. "I wish I were at County; at least I do all the operating. I can't do another month of this."

I considered sending Corey for a psych consult. No one *wants* to go back to County.

Corey thought he'd "pissed off enough doctors" that if they got together they could decide to kick him out. He hoped his ABSITE exam score was good enough to offset this offense when the word reached Dr. Organ.

Corey blew everything out of proportion. He and John were the golden boys of the residency. The idea of Dr. Organ making the smartest chief stay for extra training seemed ludicrous. But numerous stories circled how Dr. Clamp-whacker singlehandedly got residents fired after minor altercations. No trial, no discussion. Who would believe a resident over a "respectable" attending?

I didn't have a good answer for Corey, so I told him the thought I had when I was paged to pick up sandwiches for the surgeons in OR #4. "When you're feeling worthless, remember one thing: You are the sperm that won. No one can take away that victory."

"Thanks, man." He cracked a little smile.

*

Meanwhile, Dhara's grandfather died. Her contract stated that she would be granted family leave for such a situation if she arranged for any missed call to be covered. None of the other residents in her program would cover her call. She didn't go to the funeral.

In other news, surgeons are confused as to why fewer and fewer medical students are applying for general surgical residency positions.

Chapter 57

It would have been my first entire day off in 46 days. But Reed decided he needed my help. Oh well, there were only 99 days left.

I fell asleep at the nurses' station with my pen in hand as I tried to write the notes on my patient. A nurse interrupted me from my dreams by repeating "Good morning" to me an unknown number of times. After I finished the note I crawled into an empty ICU bed to wait for Brad.

I struggled to remain compassionate while so fatigued. A mother worried because her daughter felt nauseated. I initially thought, So what? Who cares? It's just some nausea—she's fine. Maybe she'll puke and feel "all better." A well-rested individual would have felt guilty for having such thoughts. If it had only taken a night without sleep to make me feel like this, what would five years of this program do? They were creating monsters.

Brad found me in the ICU bed. "You look beat. I bet that's the last time you smiled." He pointed to my badge. That's the same thing the shark-attack nec fasc guy said 8 months ago.

"I've been feeling run down, like I have the start of a sore throat. If I could have a couple nights of good sleep, I would get better."

"That's what I've felt like for the last seven years. Welcome to General Surgery."

The butt-and-gut fraternity was not exciting enough to warrant such a hazing. Of course, there was nothing new about people allowing themselves to be tortured to join an exclusive club of idiots that had gone through the same torture years before.

I decided I didn't care about the busy work, degradation, and abuse. However, I wanted to submit a request to have my sleep refunded. Those hours should have been mine. I wanted them back.

"Dr. Harrington says he doesn't like the way you write notes," Brad told me.

I asked how I should change them.

"I don't know, he was just grumbling about it."

Evan looked up from the note he was writing. "That guy complains every morning that the sun rises in the east."

Evan was always in the right place at the right time for me. He was my "self-help" guru. He advised me to stop by my house to say hello to

257

my stuff on the way home from the satellite hospital. "That's what I do; it's the price they pay for making you go over there."

"But you have a wife and kid."

"I'm sure you have something at home that you like more than being at the hospital," he grinned.

I wondered if Corey had told him I had an inflatable sex doll to substitute for Rachel. It was that sort of grin. But that's how Evan always grinned. I wished I could hang out with him more, but between our schedules and his family...

At least I'd still be hanging out with Corey for the rest of the year. The attendings had their secret meeting and decided to keep him and Dr. Landa away from each other.

When it came time for M&M there weren't any cases to report. The ones Corey mentioned had simply vanished.

I realized why surgeons were so reluctant to admit error. To admit one mistake would allow all their actions to be scrutinized for mistakes.

So, surgeons were safer if they had a God complex; to be better than everyone else and admit no error. Isn't that what patients wanted? God to be their doctor? Given a choice, wouldn't you want God to operate on you instead of a mere mortal? Mere mortals could make mistakes, but God? God was infallible. Yeah, you wanted your surgeon to be God.

And if he wasn't God, you wanted to punish him for it.

Complication?

Lawsuit!

I hoped I would never make a mistake. That way I would always be able to claim I took responsibility for my errors.

My hopes would be fulfilled for less than 24 hours.

Chapter 58

Dr. Organ made me present at Grand Rounds again. A little talk on second messengers, so drab I need not explain it. But, I had more confidence than ever. I stammered once during the opening, but then reminded myself that it was no big deal. I knew what I wanted to say, so I figured I might as well start the sentence over and say it right. Forget this medicine thing; I was going to be a public speaker. Or better, a politician. Then I could really help people.

That was where the good day ended.

A patient had an abdominal drain, which was a fenestrated plastic tube used to drain fluid from the abdominal cavity. The external end was attached to a suction bulb. What that bulb filled with revealed if there was bleeding or leaking at the surgical site. We pulled them out after a few days. But when I released the suction, cut the suture, and pulled, I only got half a drain.

I swallowed my gulp and made a conscious effort to keep my eyelids in a normal position. I'm a crappy poker player and the patient had a well-documented anxiety disorder. He had proved it to me over and over. On morning rounds he had insisted I change his IV bag because the nurse had given him a bad bag. This wasn't going to ease him.

I tried to pretend I was about to say the blandest sentence in the world. Something along the lines of my shoelace is untied so I am going to tie it. "Sir, the end of the drain usually doesn't look like this. I am going to get an x-ray of your stomach to make sure that there isn't part of it left under your skin."

"Okay, doc." He fell for it without freaking out. I placed the drain in the sink and wrote for a stat abdominal x-ray.

I am screwed. They are going to think I accidentally cut it. They're going to call me The Drainbreaker. This guy's going to have to have another surgery. He'll be here three extra days. His wound will probably get infected and I'll be presenting it at M&M. And next time a patient needs a drain removed, the attending will want to be there to examine my technique.

Crap!

And if things got really messed up, this could be a lawsuit. All because fate dealt me a bad hand. My defense would be centered upon the randomness of the universe…

Actually, Your Honor, it was inevitable that a mistake would happen. Members of the Jury, if you play the game long enough you will eventually fumble the ball. It's not my fault. It's destiny. In closing, I'd like to say two words: chaos theory. Thank you, no further arguments.

I ran to find Barclay, my rarely seen junior. She chortled enthusiastically—a welcome relief from her bitterness, even if her laughter was at my expense. And when she was done giggling she muttered, "I'm so glad it was you." Nice.

We went back to his room and prodded the wound with a forceps. He winced. She didn't feel the drain at the edge of the fascia. She went to find Dr. Kudrow, our attending. I was to "birddog" the x-ray. Birddog? She sounded like Franklin, which only added nausea on top of the sinking feeling I had in my stomach.

As I waited, I imagined the curse words Dr. Kudrow would be muttering under his breath. It didn't help that I had a suture pull out during our case the day before. Having a suture pull out during the case gave me the same feeling I had after dribbling the basketball off my leg during a fast break in sixth grade. Dr. Kudrow just gave me a disappointed look, which let my imagination say more than he possibly could have. Now I was a complete buffoon in his eyes.

I didn't worry about the patient; he just had a piece of rubber floating around his abdomen. No, I was scared for me. Kudrow seemed nice, but they all seemed nice until they bite. Kudrow was even soft-spoken. And he had fuzzy hair. Small guys with fuzzy hair don't shove their size 9s up people's butts. Right?

Barclay told me that at first he asked what I had done, like if I had forgotten to cut the suture. But she assured him I already felt guilty even though she thought it wasn't my fault. Despite laughing at me, she was at least trying to protect me.

The film showed a drain lying across the inside of the abdomen. We had to take the patient to the OR and reopen his healing midline incision. We fished out the loose drain tip.

The weight of the world slid off my shoulders when Kudrow saw that the drain had separated at the joint between the tube and the fenestrated section. My name would not become an eponym for a broken drain. Don't pull an Iaquinta when you take out that drain.

Kudrow continued, "When I walked into the room, this man was calm. I don't know what you said or how you phrased it, but I was impressed he wasn't crawling up the walls. I mean that as a compliment to you."

What a nice guy! Corey said it on the first day: "If you expect the worst, you might find yourself pleasantly surprised."

I called Rachel to fill her in on the day's events. She waited out my story and then broke her own news.

"One of the ENT interns is leaving. There's going to be a spot open!" she told me.

Having learned from my previous mistake, I tried not to diffuse the excitement. "Wow. Why, how?"

"He wants to be closer to home or something. It came to me through the grapevine. This might be our chance."

It was. I might be skeptical about God, but I believe in divine intervention...or Karma. The fact that an ENT position opened up in itself is rare, but in Madison of all places, uncanny.

"I still have the Chairman's email. I'll find out if they've opened a spot."

After we hung up I was dumbfounded. Never before had my road through life have such a widespread fork. I left Wisconsin to find my way in the world. No help. No local family or friends. And now the very place I escaped had a spot for me. I now had a path back to Wisconsin where Rachel, my family, an ENT residency, and frozen custard all waited.

On the other hand, I had committed to the position here. I hadn't even given them a chance yet. And this place was my first pick. When I left the interview a year and a half ago I had a gut feeling that this was where I belonged. Could I ignore that? I always trust my gut.

Four years in Wisconsin (more likely with Rachel) or four years in California (unlikely with Rachel)?

This would take more than a coin toss.

Chapter 59

I worked with The Organizer again. He still had plenty of rips and quips in his armamentarium. When the anesthetist asked for a time estimate, he replied, "It depends how well my opponent works against me," nodding to me. He criticized my way of tying "Christmas bows" with the suture, and told me to "tuck in my scrubs so I don't look like a butcher," a distinct departure from his father's janitor comment.

I hoped that by fulfilling his verbal abuse quota at work, he would go home with nothing but nice things to say to his family. I just kept my mouth shut and watched. I took in some of his techniques, but I also went through the powers of 2 in my head. 2^{20} equals 1,048,576. I think. I'm one of five people in the world that believes there is something relaxing about math.

Then, I got to work with Dr. Hou. No, not Who. She's a plastic surgeon. I assisted her on a bilateral breast reduction. Did you know that outside of the age range of 20 to 30, more women get breast reductions than implants? (Maybe not in L.A.).

Just like The Organizer, she had her own set of rules to be followed. Barclay warned me to meet her well before the case and not to say or do anything unless told. Barclay made Dr. Hou seem more intimidating than The Organizer. The latter was predictable—any movement, wrong or otherwise, would initiate a string of insults; but he didn't eject people from the game. Dr. Hou kicked Brad out of the OR because he didn't properly introduce himself. She sounded like a ticking bomb. Oh well, I'd just spent the last 2^8 (256) days working with difficult people; I could take whatever she dished out.

I arrived to the Pre-Op holding area before Dr. Hou and her patient. There would be no surprise introduction seconds before the case started. If she needed 10 minutes to pimp me, I'd be there for eleven. Like a good intern, I was punctual and my teeth were brushed.

I steeled myself for anything, but Dr. Hou still took me off guard. I couldn't remain frightened of an Asian woman with soft features and pep in her voice. Maybe that was part of her modus operandi, disarm with kindness and then go for the kill.

As soon as the patient was asleep, Dr. Hou stripped off the patient's gown. Ink lines crossed the patient's breast like her skin was a sewing pattern. Dr. Hou drew them when the patient was upright so she could see how gravity affected the breasts. She looked at them for a moment like a contractor looking at blueprints and then turned to me and said, "I read your file, so I know it will be worth my time to teach you the Art of Surgery."

I almost passed out for the second time that year. What? Read my file? Wanted to teach? What a difference from Dr. Fagan, who merely said "Oh" and thought all learning should occur via book on my own time.

She didn't want me to learn how to do a breast reduction; she already knew that wasn't in my future. She wanted me to learn the concepts. The breast is a somewhat spherical object; to decrease its size but still have the nipple in the proper position, the skin taut, and a normal contour was a lesson in geometry and tailoring. We didn't want the patient to end up with "stargazers" (nipples looking into space). I liked her slang. I hesitated telling her about "Cleveland nipple," which is when one nipple looks at you and the other looks at Cleveland.

Once she saw my interest in learning, the floodgates opened. A breast reduction takes a few hours. We interspersed conversations about cooking and art in with teaching and quiz sessions. For the first time all year, an attending surgeon interacted with me like I was a real human.

By the end of the case, I knew I loved her. See how susceptible residents are? One person treats us kindly for a few hours and we think we are in love.

Chapter 60

The real love of my life was waiting to hear about my potential transfer. The ENT program definitely had a spot available. Applications were due immediately and as soon as they found a good candidate they'd fill the spot. No crazy match program.

I had a good chance of getting the spot. The doctors there knew me from my medical school rotations. If only I could say I really wanted it.

It had nothing to do with Rachel and I had no way of explaining it to her in a way she'd believe. I had committed to five years in Oakland. That's it. In my opinion, almost nothing should break that deal. Leaving them in the lurch wouldn't be polite.

But in Rachel's eyes I'd be choosing Oakland over her. I suppose it looked that simple. I could hear the voices in my head: "If you truly loved her, there wouldn't be a decision."

If that were true, then the fact that I debated what to do could only mean I didn't love her enough. But that didn't feel like the truth either.

Couldn't I just have a teleporter? Life is so unfair.

Moving to California was the first real thing I had ever done. As a high-schooler, I had only applied to one college. And I didn't even apply to any other medical schools. I never lived more than an hour and forty-five minutes from home. That's what I tried to explain to Rachel. Oakland represented me going out in the world and grabbing it by the tail and wrestling it to the ground.

I told her that I was nearing the end of a tunnel and that I'd soon be in the big bright light. I couldn't click my heels and go home, not now. Maybe not ever.

She observed that if we didn't get together now, there would be no reasonable expectation that anything would change in the next two years.

Chapter 61

My first day off in fifty-nine days! I woke up at 5:30 a.m. but I told myself I deserved to sleep in. I owed my body. So, I got up at 6:30 a.m. How refreshing.

As I cleaned my apartment, my phone rang.

"Hello?"

"Sal?"

"Yeah," I recognized the voice.

"It's Brad. I figured you were awake by now, relaxing in your pad. I got a question for you. Do you know about patient Wilson?"

I didn't.

"Are you sure? I've got Dr. Harrington breathing down my neck right now because no one saw her yesterday and none of us seem to know about her."

"Who is she?"

"She's a patient of Dr. Harrington's that had a wound dehiscence. The admit orders say Team Three is aware. But no one told me and Barclay was gone."

Crap. They did it to us again. For the second time, they admitted a patient to our service without telling us.

"I haven't heard of her."

"Are you sure?"

"I don't lie. Who wrote the admit orders?"

"I don't know, I can't read their signature." That limited it to half the surgery residents.

I sighed.

"Hey, I'm fucking with you. I just wanted to harass you one last time. See if I could get you riled up."

I chuckled.

"It was fun working with you. Great job."

Very funny, razzing the intern at 7 a.m. on his day off.

Part 6: THE BURN UNIT

Chapter 62

The Burn Hospital was actually two neighboring hospitals, UC Davis and Shriners (for the kids). It was over an hour from my place in Oakland, but they had a place for me to stay within the university hospital. I was excited when one of the program coordinators said, "You'll be staying in one of the new call rooms." I envisioned a TV and VCR, maybe a computer, or some of those exotic women fanning me with palm leaves and feeding me grapes.

The correct interpretation of "new call room" is actually "a room that's been newly designated as a call room." My room was a barely remodeled patient room. I thought the "sharps disposal" unit and the oxygen hook-up on the wall were novel amenities, but where was I going to shower?

I worked with two attendings and two residents from the UC Davis general surgery program. Sandy, a junior, was the acting chief of the service. She was a twig. She pulled her hair back into a pigtail, which made her look fifteen. At first, I thought Sandy was one of those rare happy residents, not worn down by three years of general surgery. She quickly confessed that she was just happy to be on Burns because it was a "cake" rotation.

Sandy handed me a pager that morning. Of course they give you call on your first day.

"What's this?" I already had a pager on my hip.

"It's the code pager for the children's hospital."

I dreaded that idea. I had given CPR to a dying baby once. Something I hoped to never do again. But Sandy assured me that the thing never goes off. The children's unit had only ever had five codes.

A pessimist knows when he just got jinxed.

So, I walked around with two pagers on my hip. Boy, did I look important! Everything was great, for about two hours.

Then, the code pager went off. What in Sam Hill was going on here! Five codes ever and I couldn't hold the pager for two hours? I wanted to toss the pager into the closest garbage can and casually walk away. Ho hum, nothing going on here. Whistle, whistle.

I answered the page.

"Hello, this is the page operator."

"Yes, I am answering for 55992."

"Good morning, that was a test page. Just making sure the system works."

"Do you do that often?"

"Every morning."

Whew.

Thanks, Sandy. Now I have to go to the ER to get treated for my heart attack.

*

Clinic proved to me that all kids were trying to kill themselves. Boiling pots of water, barbecue grills, rice cookers, kerosene lamps, and campfires. I didn't understand why all parents weren't freaks. One little girl had been burnt in the face and chest. Her lips could hardly smile through her melted, wrinkled face. But her eyes shone and her voice sounded as sweet as a little girl's could be. She remained a cutie underneath all those scars, but how many other people would be able to see that? What did the kids at school say? Did she go to a regular school? What would she be like ten years from now?

There were no burn victim admissions that night, but that was not to say call was uneventful. First, I got a parking ticket. What a waste of precious money. I had parked in the wrong visitor lot.

Then, for the second time in my short medical career, I tripped the fire alarm in a stairwell. I am not observant enough for some stairwells to be passable and others to be for emergency only. If I were lazy enough to take the elevator, this wouldn't happen. But then how would the nurses have gotten their laughs that night?

Being smart enough to be a doctor in no way implies I am smart enough to read the signs that tell me where to park or which doors not to open. I take comfort in that absentmindedness can be endearing.

They let me stay in the Pediatric Burns call room. That room was the lap of luxury compared to the cell they detained me in the other nights. Not only did it have a shower, but also a TV and VCR. Someone must have been toying with me. The bed was also comfortable, and I didn't mean in comparison to hospital beds, I meant in comparison to all beds. Didn't they know they were risking me actually falling asleep on call? I was sure someone had lost his or her job over that blunder. Comfy beds? Next we'd want shorter work hours.

A spastic nurse did her best to keep me from sleeping in that fine bed. She had numerous concerns, but only half of them valid. I explained my point of view and gave her verbal orders. What she didn't tell me was that she disagreed with all of my decisions. So, she called my attending at 2:45 a.m.

My blood pressure skyrocketed when I found out the next morning. She had set me up. She put me at the attending's mercy. I confronted her on it.

"From now on, if you disagree with my treatment plan, or have questions regarding it, I would be happy to discuss it. I think it is unnecessary for you to wake up my attending before our discussion is finished."

"I thought we were done."

"You gave me no indication that you disagreed with my plan."

"Well, I know how they work you guys, you're covering two hospitals... they work you over." How could she think she had done me a favor? Didn't she know attendings breathed fire?

"That's all right." I backed down. "From now on just page me if you have a question."

Sandy confirmed that the nurses were aggressive in getting their plan followed. She said one had even called Dr. Silva, our attending burn surgeon of the month, telling him the patient needed fasciotomies and then proceeded to slit the man's legs open before Dr. Silva showed up.

Maybe The Organism had jokingly stated the truth when he called me his opponent. I found it hard to believe we were a health care "team."

*

Severe burn patients lack a place to start an IV. I couldn't find a vein on an arm that looked like a burnt hot dog. A central line remained the only option. These lines entered the major blood vessels of the body; the femoral vein, the jugular vein, or the subclavian vein.

One of my goals of the year was to not stick myself. They say "everyone gets stuck," but I didn't want to be everyone. However, after inserting a line into a man's femoral vein, I proceeded to stick the needle into my hand.

I had visions of HIV and hepatitis C viruses scrambling to get into my bloodstream. I stopped everything to go wash my hands. I remembered Corey's statement: The patient can die as long as we don't get HIV.

I filled out forms in triplicate describing the incident. Under sterile technique I poked my finger with a needle that had entered the patient's skin. I went to the lab to have my blood drawn. I had to prove I wasn't already infected. Then, I wrote orders for the patient's blood to be drawn. In six weeks they would draw my blood again to see if I had contracted anything. I hoped that the man would have negative blood work. That would ease my worry.

I had recently read a story about a nurse who had contracted hepatitis C and needed a liver transplant. She was only in her forties. The last thing I needed was that thought lingering in the back of my mind for the next six weeks on top of everything else.

*

Another bit of medical advice:

Don't put a lit blowtorch in your back pocket.

It actually happened to a man who thought he turned the torch off. Burnt butts aren't pretty.

Chapter 63

I lived the first 25 years of my life without knowing that people frequently try to commit suicide by burning themselves to death. Didn't people know of less painful ways to go? There needed to be a Government Task Force to get the word out. There could be a poster contest for grade school kids. How about a guy hanging in a noose and the caption "Not as Messy as Burning Yourself to Death"?

One man on our service tried to commit suicide by driving into a wall. His car had caught fire and he was burned across the neck, chest, and abdomen. That morning. we debrided his burns and skin-grafted him.

I had grafted skin before, but nothing like this. Third-degree burns needed to be fully excised. Third-degree means the skin, or even deeper, is dead. (First degree is just the outer layer of skin. Second degree includes damage to deeper skin—blistering occurs). Treatment requires removing strips of skin like you're the Greek guy carving off meat for gyros. We had to keep removing strips of skin until we got to live, bleeding tissue. A graft will only live on bleeding tissue. Extensively burned patients lose a lot of skin. Skin loss equals heat loss; skin regulates body temperature. So, for big burn cases we cranked the room temperature up into the nineties. Putting on a cloth gown and double gloves (now that I had learned my lesson the hard way, I always double gloved) brought back memories of passing out. They kept Gatorade in the OR in case we got dehydrated during a long case.

I operated with Dr. Silva for the first time. We hacked out pieces of burn the size of salad plates from the abdomen of a badly burnt man. I wished I owned a knife like the one we used. I would have amazed John at his turkey dinner. The knife looked like a cellist's bow, but with a guard like a razor.

Dr. Silva taught me to play the wound like a violin. I fiddled across the width of the wound while slowly advancing. I lifted great hunks of flesh off in sheets, like shaving cheese. When the dead tissue didn't bleed after my first pass, Dr. Silva ordered me to take more, just like my grandma would at Thanksgiving. After the third pass, I had removed all the thickened skin, leaving only subcutaneous fat.

Human fat is just like chicken fat, yellow and slimy. It pulls apart. It coats the instruments and the gloves and gives you "butterfingers."

Dr. Silva wasn't used to me, so I spared him from the jokes that must have been said a thousand times over. That didn't keep me from thinking about "slap me some skin" and "no skin off my back" and "there's more than one way to skin a cat." Trying to stifle giggles doesn't help keep body temperature down.

*

That night on call, I admitted yet another child with a scald burn. He had been "helping" his dad make macaroni. While his dad talked on the phone, he reached up, grabbed the pot, and tried to pour its contents into the colander in the sink. Instead, it toppled backwards and spilled down his face onto his chest and belly.

I wonder what the person on the other end of the phone thought as he heard the sudden screaming of the six-year-old.

Dad told me his son "never did anything like this before."

Of course not, because if he did and you let him burn himself again I'd be calling Social Services. It seemed near negligence just to have created the situation where his son could pull the boiling pot off of the stove.

That being said, I am sure an ER doctor out there would argue that my mom had committed negligence, too. Despite her best attempts to save me from myself, I still broke an arm roller-skating, split my knee open on the playground, dislocated my shoulder playing basketball, and had the back of my scalp split open by a friend.

But burns seemed more avoidable. There was only one hot thing; just keep the kid away from it. And keep your hot water heater set at 120 degrees. Hotter temperatures burn infants faster than you can get them out of the water. A baby's skin is thinner and more sensitive. And why should your shower water get so hot it could scald you?

*

I called Rachel to share the horrors of the burn unit with her. I also told her that a friend of mine had been diagnosed with celiac sprue.

"Wow, that's rare. We just learned about that in GI."

"Yeah, she said she heard about it and it sounded exactly like her digestive problems, so she got tested and it turned out positive." Celiac disease is a digestive intolerance to gluten, which is in any wheat or rye product.

"Which friend?" Rachel asked.

"Oh, no one you know."

271

But she wanted to know who.

"I think I shouldn't say. I don't want to disclose healthcare information."

"Please." Her sarcasm reached through the phone and snapped my ear.

"What difference does it make?"

"Exactly, no difference. I don't know her, so why can't you tell me her name?"

"I think I should just assume privacy." Some people are private about their health. I am.

"You don't trust me enough to tell me her name?" I heard the disappointment in her voice. "I'm not going to tell the world your friend has celiac disease."

I didn't want to argue this. "It has nothing to do with you. I just think I should assume it's not okay to pass gossip like that."

"People assume that any secrets they tell someone will be shared with their significant other, but that it will go no further," she argued.

"But what about the principle?"

"What about trusting me?"

"What about keeping the trust of the person who told me the information?"

Rachel called it what it was. "I give up. My point doesn't matter. Even if you agreed with what I'm saying, you are too stubborn to change your mind."

"Do you want to talk about something else?" I offered.

"No."

After she hung up, I went to the bathroom. My reflection in the mirror rolled his eyes at me.

Why did you make the wrong choice?

Come on! You're not on her side, are you? Doesn't anyone in this world care about principle?

Yes, but care about principle when principle matters.

You know, you've got a slender neck. I bet you'd be easy to trach.

272

Chapter 64

That day, Dr. Silva and I admitted another child. Dr. Silva had an air of informality about him, like what he was doing was equivalent to fixing your toilet. We'll just need to excise that and cover it with a graft from the other thigh. He looked like a plumber, too. He had glasses, a salt-and-pepper bushy mustache, and matching hair that would have best been contained under a baseball cap. A T-shirt would have fit him better than a shirt and tie.

The patient's grandmother had spilt hot water on her while they were cooking in the kitchen.

I was wrong. It wasn't bad parenting. These parents feel like the worst parents in the world (if they didn't I got suspicious). I realized that little kids had a death wish, but we politely called it curiosity. Another kid managed to pry open a thermos and spill its scalding contents onto his feet. He needed a skin graft.

I asked Dr. Silva if he ever got sick of hearing these stories.

"Yeah, and I've heard some dumb ones."

I wanted to hear them.

"One night a guy was driving and he ran out of gas. But he couldn't believe it, so he opened up the gas tank on his car and tried to see inside the tank by lighting a match."

"No way!"

"Actually, I've had that one happen twice. Or, how about this? One woman decided to kill her little girl's lice with gasoline. So, she started washing her daughter's hair with gasoline while she smoked a cigarette. That girl needed her entire scalp and the back of her neck grafted."

That evening when I called Rachel, she didn't waste time getting to what was on her mind. "I thought about the conversation we had the other night. You know, the one where you wouldn't tell me who had celiac disease. I think that was the last straw."

After my heart crawled back up from my stomach and started pumping blood, I thought last straw? What about the other straws? Nobody told me I was on my last-ups. You never called out "Uno."

"What do you mean, last straw?" I asked.

"I don't know how compatible we are. I think you might have schizoid personality disorder."

Obviously the GI rotation was over and now she was onto psychiatry. Nothing refreshes a relationship like diagnosing a personality disorder in your loved one. Schizoid personality was not schizophrenia. It described an introvert with few close friends besides family members. Furthermore, schizoids didn't care what other people thought about them or their actions. I sort of fit the bill, but when it came down to the actual criteria I think I would argue a little harder. But, in a moment of clarity, I knew that discussing the accuracy of her diagnosis was not the heart of the matter.

"Another thing, I think it is highly unlikely that you will ever take dance lessons and go dancing with me."

"I can't dispute that." I looked dumbly at my feet. I had not been aware how important this was to her.

"And your baseline is sad. You need a reason to be happy whereas I am the opposite. Have you ever thought about anti-depressants?"

"Those things are just sugar pills anyway." I think there's a difference between sarcastic and depressed. And I think working over 130 hours a week might not have allowed me to be the person I really am. Of course, the real me wasn't a dancer either.

She didn't find that funny. "You don't disclose enough of your personal feelings. You're very good at making little jokes and evading talking about yourself."

Crap, she had me there. Just a few days earlier Corey had asked why I always talked about my mom but never mentioned my dad. I had known Corey for nine months and he had just found out that my dad had passed away.

The conversation actually became less of a conversation and more of a listing of my faults. I didn't have anything to say. I hadn't recovered from the words "last straw."

Why hadn't she pointed out these faults all along?

The last time I had this feeling, I was delivering CPR to a dying woman.

I sat silent on the other end of the line. I couldn't argue her feelings. If I didn't disclose enough to her, if I scraped the cookie dough bowl too much, if I insulted her ability to make a decision about moving out here, my intention didn't matter. She was insulted. What could I do?

"I'm sorry...but look on the bright side, at least I'm not Charles Manson." A little optimism might cheer her up.

"You're doing it. NO little jokes."

C'mon, that's all I got. It's what I am. I can't take anything seriously. Life is but a dream.

I disagreed that our relationship was unhealthy. Distance divided us, but that was an external factor. When we were together there wasn't any stress. If she could leave me to myself to fall down the mountain while learning to snowboard, things were fine.

The fact that I didn't disclose my secrets or feelings troubled me. Not because I held them back, but because I felt like I had nothing to hold back. I wondered if real humans had more complex feelings than me. Things are what they are. I didn't silently ruminate feelings. I ruminated about letters, numbers, and shapes. I had recently figured out that the word "sedative" can be rearranged to "deviates" but that didn't excite her, or anyone else on the planet, so I kept that to myself.

I concluded two things. If I started drinking I could probably get loose enough to dance. And, although she was not happy, I didn't want to give up...even if for the selfish reason that she was my life-preserver of sanity.

Instead of falling asleep I tried to solve our relationship. It presented quite a conundrum. I thought actions, not words, define a person. Yet I could only use words from my prison-cell-call-room to prove anything to her. But I was soon interrupted. A transfer from another hospital arrived.

Mr. Haines, at the age of 94, had been riding his ATV and tipped it over into a brush fire. He had intended on parking near the fire, but instead fell into it.

Third-degree burns covered his right leg and both hands. He didn't have pain because he had fried the nerves. His face glowed red with second-degree burns. A sharp stripe of normal forehead demarcated where his hat had been.

His feet hung off the gurney. I estimated he'd stand about six-four. And he sat straight, not hunched over like so many elderly people get. If I didn't know his age, I would have guessed seventy-five.

"Hi-ya, Doc," he chimed as I approached.

He remained perky throughout the exam. The ninety-year-olds I met tended to be quite alert. When people got to be that age, it was because they didn't have serious health problems. Granted, he had two pacemakers (the first one had failed), but that paled in comparison to having diabetes. I'd never met a ninety-year-old diabetic. I noticed that he had partial amputations of the fourth and fifth fingers of his right hand.

He told me lost those fingers a few years earlier in a sawmill accident.

A few years ago? "Ten, twenty years ago?"

"No, a few years ago. Say, is this going to take very long? I've got to finish burning my brush piles while the weather is good."

I doubted I would live until I was ninety, and this guy had worked in a sawmill a few years ago. Incredible. A few days earlier I had seen a 76-year-old who burned his hand while using an acetylene torch to fix his Model-T Ford. That guy had been a spring chicken compared to this one. But they both had the same attitude, the how-much-longer-before-I-can-leave-because-I've-got-projects-I-am-working-on attitude.

I didn't mind staying up to care for him. I couldn't sleep anyway. Snippets of Rachel's words chased each other around in my mind. When I finally dozed off at 5 a.m., I dreamt I had a burn on my face and my lip wouldn't move.

Rachel hadn't played fair. You can't let it all build up until you explode. If those things bothered her, she should have told me.

*

That next morning Rachel and I talked again. I told her what I felt.

"If you don't think this relationship is going anywhere, I think we should wait before breaking up. I'm not ready to stop now. I enjoy dating you too much." But if she slowly became a creep over the next couple of months then I'd be glad to rid myself of her. She'd do that for me if I asked.

We talked about when we would see each other next, and what I would do during my week off at the end of internship. I told her I would be going to a friend's wedding that week.

"Have you thought about seeing anyone?" she asked.

"Oh, I have some other friends that I will catch up with, too."

She laughed. "Actually, I was talking about seeing a psychiatrist."

"Oh, that. No. You want me to get on Zoloft right away so I will be happy the next time you come and visit? Maybe I will be so happy that I'll be dancing on the tables. Everything will be cured at once."

She laughed. See, I still could make jokes at a serious question to turn the focus elsewhere.

Chapter 65

I missed Easter Sunday dinner at John's house because I was on call. But, I couldn't have asked for a nicer day. I sat outside and read in the sun. Dr. Silva had warned me that every year some elderly woman bent over to pull the heavy ham out of the oven and accidentally dumped it onto her feet. Then, she slipped on the scalding oil and fell on her butt, right into the boiling juices.

But that didn't happen. Nothing happened.

The next morning in clinic I saw a man that had 40% TBSA (total body surface-area burns). He had been grafted the previous summer. His grafted skin looked like that of an action figure's that had been left out in the sun on a hot day. His "friends" had doused him with gasoline and lit him on fire after a drug deal had gone bad.

Why, people, why? Why must you hurt each other?

Why, Rachel, why must we hurt each other?

I noticed that my problems with Rachel hadn't started until I had met Dhara. But I barely saw or talked to Dhara because of our all-encompassing jobs. However, if you'll recall, Dhara hadn't even made Rachel's laundry list of my faults. I had supplied enough ammo on my own.

When Rachel and I talked that evening, everything seemed like old times. We took a break from scrutinizing my faults to joke around. I tried to convince her that if I were a fun-loving, extroverted, dancer-guy soon every woman would be throwing herself at me.

I wasn't sure she bought it.

Chapter 66

That morning Sandy commented on how quiet the service had been.

I rapidly knocked on wood and held my index finger to my lips. We all knew we hadn't had any major admissions for weeks. Her saying it out loud jinxed us.

She ignored my cue to shut-up. "Do you know what we haven't had? Meth lab explosions."

"Meth lab explosions?"

She explained that there were quite a few meth labs in the area. People set up labs in their basements and worked in Speedos because the labs were super hot from the chemical reactions. They came in with 95% TBSA burns with a little Speedo outline of normal skin. That meant that all the skin grafts had to be harvested from the butt to recover the damaged areas.

How cruel. Someone out there was literally an assface.

*

A ruddy man in his mid-forties wearing an old flannel shirt arrived at midnight with burns on his hands and thighs. He said he had met up with an old army buddy at the convenience mart and gone to his house. They were in the garage when he lit a cigarette and something blew up, catching his pants on fire.

The paramedics found a handgun on him. This aroused the policemen. Seriously, concealed weapons give them erections. An officer asked Mr. Doe, "Did you know the gun you were carrying had the serial number scratched off of it?"

"Yes, that's why I was going to get rid of it." The perks of this job are incredible.

"Did this friend of yours have chemicals in his garage? Were there any test tubes or flasks of chemicals around?" the boyish officer asked. Policemen are always so young.

"No."

The cops left. Sandy and I tended to Mr. Doe's wounds. A nurse administered morphine into his IV.

"That story I just told wasn't the truth," he confessed.

"What is the truth?" Sandy asked. It sounded like a deep question.

"We weren't in the garage. We were in the kitchen."

It still didn't make sense. Something really burned him.

Then the morphine kicked in. Sandy and I weren't aware that high doses of morphine inspire truth-telling. This might be a worthwhile case report.

"Go get the police officer," he asked drowsily.

"You are about to fall asleep, Mr. Doe," Sandy said.

"I know, that is why you need to get him. I feel like telling the truth before I fall asleep."

The "truth" was that he drove from Nevada to pick up supplies for making meth-amphetamine. Someone had paid him $1600 for this mission. Then, Someone told him that if he lit red phosphorus on a piece of metal it would burn a hole in the metal.

Mr. Doe lit the red phosphorus on a piece of metal he held in his hands. The red phosphorus exploded, catching his pants on fire. Then, he beat out the fire with his hands.

I sent Sandy to go work for the Psychic Friends Network.

*

After midnight, I realized I had just started day 300. Yes. They couldn't stop the clock.

Chapter 67

Rachel had more bad news for me. She had talked to a couple of epidemiologists and they both recommended that she not do her Masters during medical school. If she ended up at the CDC, they would arrange for her to get her Masters.

That solidified the idea that there was no chance of us being together in the next two years. The most she could do is take a couple of rotations out here as a fourth year medical student. We would have to make a big decision.

I told Rachel, "If you decide to break up with me, don't do it until June first."

"Why?"

"So, we don't have to worry about anything awkward when you visit at the end of May. You already bought the tickets."

"You just don't want to break up so we can have sex."

"No, that's not true. I'd want to have sex with you even if you dumped me."

*

The thought of losing Rachel depressed me, but the next admission outright broke my heart. A single man and his two children had been caught in a house fire. The man had rescued his five-year-old son without injury and then went back for his daughter. By the time he reemerged, the three-year-old had suffered 93% TBSA and he suffered 100% TBSA as well as injuries.

I could hardly recognize her as human. Black skin covered her from head to toe minus a small patch of skin on her scalp extending onto the back of her neck. She came intubated but we put in some more lines. Then Dr. Silva and I performed escharotomies, scar incisions. We cut both legs from hips to toes, across her abdomen and chest, and down the lengths of her arms. We even filleted her eyelids open. These incisions prevented the swelling from building up pressure under the charred skin and thereby cutting off the blood supply and return flow. Her fingers had already split open by themselves due to the burnt skin and swelling. She would be lucky if she kept any of her fingers. She would be lucky if she lived at all. Or maybe she would be unlucky to live.

Tomorrow we'd cut off all of her dead skin and cover her in

synthetic skin because she didn't have any donor areas. That is, if she survived the night. We didn't know the extent of her lung injury.

They life-flighted the little girl to us from Mexico. The Shriners Hospital immediately accepted her because there was a fund of donated money for such specific cases. Thanks to generous people, she'd receive the best healthcare in the world.

But her father stayed behind in Mexico. He would probably die in the next few days. We couldn't offer him the healthcare his daughter would receive. If he hadn't run back into the burning house, she would have died. But his heroism didn't earn him hundreds of thousands of dollars in healthcare.

How could we have made this choice? First, how did we choose a child over a young adult? How do we choose to spend hundreds of thousands on one child with a poor prognosis over helping numerous children with good prognoses? And how is it we decide to go ahead and try in the worst of situations, rather than just give her palliative care?

I didn't know the answers. I felt irritated that a man who nearly sacrificed his life for his daughter wouldn't get healthcare as a reward. I felt saddened that a three-year-old girl would lose all her fingers and toes and would be covered with scars from head to toe for the rest of her life. Assuming she lived, she would always be the subject of stares and ridicule from other kids. And the scars wouldn't let her grow to a normal stature.

It was hard to feel like I was doing the right thing when I couldn't foresee an end to the suffering. But if my child were in the same position, I probably wouldn't have any questions.

*

The next morning in burn clinic I met a 13-year-old girl who looked like she was six; her scars never let her grow the way she should have. And people treated her like she was six. I had to constantly remind myself not to make the same mistake. When given a chance, she'd act like a teenager.

Although some of the children had serious psychological repercussions from their trauma, most of them were still normal people. Normal people trapped inside lousy skin. Just knowing that the little girl from Mexico could emerge from all this physical trauma with a normal psyche offset many of my previous concerns.

*

We brought the little girl back to the OR to remove more dead tissue and cover her with grafts. We unwrapped her like a little mummy. By the time we finished debriding the burnt skin from her tiny arms and legs, we had removed all of her skin. Her fingers were lifeless blackened stubs. I couldn't tell if it was my imagination or if she really smelled like smoke. I was too embarrassed to ask.

Dr. Silva said her fingers would have to be cut off, but he wasn't in a hurry to do it. "Maybe next week," he said. I was seeing the last of those fingers. She found the worst way to get out of piano recitals.

The dead skin of her face looked like the belly of a bloated toad. The pink flesh of her eyelids bulged through the escharotomy incisions. Her lips glistened like fat red sausages. When I steadied her head, my fingers sank into the gray, puffy skin of her bloated head like she was a rotten pumpkin.

We harvested her only remaining good skin from her scalp. By removing a very thin layer, the skin would grow back on her scalp. We meshed the graft 4:1 with a device that puts numerous perforations in the graft. This lets is open like a fishnet, so that the area that can be covered is four times larger than the original graft. The gaps fill in once the graft "takes" to its transplanted site. While I helped Sandy finish one arm she said to me, "I thought a lot last night about what you said, about the girl being here and the father left behind. It's wrong."

It still didn't sit well with me. "At least the uncle is here. He seems to be a caring man."

Sandy agreed, but said he always stands outside the room. The morning after the fire he bought a newspaper that showed a picture of the burn victims. He was too afraid to go into the room to see the girl. That afternoon I checked on the little girl. Sure enough, her uncle was standing outside her room like a security guard. I talked to him briefly. After some small talk I asked how the dad was doing.

The uncle said his brother had died yesterday.

I felt nauseated. I could only say, "I'm sorry." I wanted someone to blame, and I wasn't even a family member. He should have been here. The outcome would have probably been the same, but that didn't matter. It was the principle, and this was one of the moments when I thought it really mattered.

The next patient we admitted might as well have been her dad. He had suffered a 94% total body surface area burn. He crashed his car and managed to roll out of it when it burst into flames. When the rescue team arrived he sat awake and alert, unaware of his prognosis.

Dr. Silva told me, "I've had patients with total body burns ask me if they were going to be all right. I've looked them right in the eye and said no." For an adult with greater than 70% TBSA burn, the odds are against survival. The only reason this man could talk was that he had only fried his skin. His body hadn't realized the extent of injury to its largest organ. Within hours we'd have to put an airway into his swelling throat and then perform escharotomies on his burnt skin.

We worked him up as a trauma patient because of the method of his injury. While the patient sat in the CT scanner, Dr. Silva noticed the song overhead on the radio: Bruce Springsteen's "I'm on Fire." The universe has a sick sense of humor.

At 3 a.m., a mother brought her three-year-old boy to the ER with scald burns to both of his feet. She tried to convince us that he had wet the bed, secretly went into bathtub to wash up, and accidentally burned his feet.

Nobody jumps into a scalding hot bathtub two feet at a time.

The most common time for "dips" was during potty training. She had punished him for wetting the bed. We immediately called Social Services.

A man had just died trying to save his daughter from a fire and in front of me was a woman who had just scalded her son as a bedwetting punishment. It really was a sick world.

That night, I finished my Burn Rotation. No wonder why Rachel thought my baseline was sad. How could anyone witness these injuries on a daily basis and remain cheerful?

Part 7: HMO Again
Chapter 68

That morning we had a late OR start so we didn't meet until 7 a.m. I sat in the resident's lounge a few minutes, wondering who was on my team. Then Beetle strolled in. A smile crept onto my face. I'd have someone to help make the best of whatever lousy situation we found ourselves in.

Beetle and I finished shooting the breeze at quarter after, but Liz, our notorious chief, still hadn't shown. But then Beetle's pager rattled.

"That's Finley, she got her eighth flat tire of the year and will be here in a little while." Liz had achieved notoriety for her "car mishaps." I'd never worked with her, but the rumor mill regularly churned out stories about her.

"Yeah," Beetle laughed.

I eavesdropped on Beetle's call. He hung up after a yeah, an oh, and an uh-huh. "That was her, all right. She's having car trouble and we should go ahead and round without her."

I chuckled.

"There is no way I am going to put up with eight weeks of that," Beetle said. It was true; for reasons unknown, I was to spend the last two months of my internship with the two of them.

I couldn't confirm that Liz ever arrived. I operated all day and when I finished she had already left for the day. One down, 53 to go.

*

The next night, while on call, Rachel paged me. If I had known that it would have been my only half-hour to get sleep I would not have called her back—for more reasons than one.

She said to me, "I've decided we should break up on June first."

"Hey, I was just kidding about that June thing. I'm not ready for that."

"Well, I've thought about it. We both agree we wouldn't want to do a long-distance relationship for two or three years. That's not a real relationship. So, that means that we have to break up. Why waste time together now if we know it is just going to end?"

Ouch. The King of Logic had gotten his heart broken by the Queen of Logic.

She got my gerbil all fired up on its wheel. Even if it wound up being a quiet night, I wouldn't have been able to slow my mind enough to sleep. Was she crazy? We were good together. Where was the real Rachel? What have you done to her?

How could Rachel be breaking up with me? I had just bought a box of condoms. How inconsiderate. If for no other reason, we should keep dating at least until the condoms were gone.

I drifted throughout the hospital the remainder of the night. I wrote orders. I admitted patients. I think I even operated. But, I only remember Rachel setting the deadline.

*

While Beetle and I rounded the next morning, he told me about working all night with Liz. "In a way she's a messenger angel, solidifying my hatred of General Surgery. She's going to make it easy for me to leave." She disappeared again for six hours that morning while Beetle and I did all the work. I wished I hadn't already wasted my "There's-No-'I'-in-Team" speech the day before.

Beetle wanted to transfer programs, but had to go where he already knew people. He wanted to get as far in as possible before asking for a letter of recommendation. He said, "If I ask the big 'O' (Dr. Organ) for a letter, I risk hanging myself. I would have to be certain another program wanted me before I did that. This is going to be ugly."

He couldn't apply to the university program in Colorado because the chair and Dr. Organ were good friends. That left him with the nearby community program. But, it turned out that the chair there had trained under Dr. Organ.

Dr. Organ was God. He seemed to have his eyes and hands everywhere.

Despite Beetle's hatred for the General Surgery program, he still kept things fun. When I reached around his back to tap him on the other shoulder, he turned that way. Then, he grinned, "Oooh, that was a good one. The tap-the-other-shoulder is one of my favorites."

*

In between cases I ran to the clinic to grab my lunch from the refrigerator. The shelves sat empty. Somebody had stolen my lunch. I was sick of being reminded that dishonest people existed in every nook of society. I didn't understand how my lunch could have tasted good to the thief. The sensation of taste obviously wasn't linked to the

286

conscience.

I wrote a note and taped it to the refrigerator. It said, "To whoever stole my lunch, I am very disappointed that my food is not safe in this refrigerator. Your thievery has left me a starving intern. I curse you. Sincerely, Sal." Didn't they know I could pass out?

By that post-call evening I was starved and spent. Liz took off to go meet some friends for a late dinner without dictating the amputation she did and without seeing the patient to the recovery room. While I cleaned up her messes, Beetle came in to say he signed out for me.

"The past forty hours are the best example of why no one should go into General Surgery. See you tomorrow morning," he said.

He disappeared out the door before I could agree.

Chapter 69

That morning when I got to the hospital, there was an overhead page for Beetle. I hadn't seen him yet so I called the page operator. She connected me to Liz.

"Where's Beetle?" she snapped.

"I haven't seen him yet, so I answered the page."

"Well have him call me on my cell as soon as he gets in." And she hung up.

A few minutes later, I ran into Beetle. "I answered your overhead page. Liz wants you to give her a call."

"Great, she's going to yell at me for not answering her page." Beetle called her. He made his way through the conversation non-verbally, then slammed the phone down. "She yelled at me for being late."

I repeated the comic scenario. "She has the gall to call you from her cell phone, from her car, to yell at *you* for being late?"

"That's just how she is. She is an idiot."

An hour later we found out that Ramirez, one of the junior residents, had just quit. He was supposed to be on call, but instead he called in and said that he wasn't coming. No, not today, nor tomorrow; never, he quit. Nobody knew what had pushed him over the edge; he seemed bitter like everyone else, but not particularly more bitter.

One of the reasons the residents were so unhappy was because we weren't from the attendings' generation. We had grown up hearing that previous generations were responsible for Vietnam and pollution and the ozone. They were greedy. They were sexist. Their marketing scams and political scandals made us skeptical of everything. We had to avoid repeating their mistakes, and fix them at the same time.

The residents had grown up with a new rulebook, but were forced to play old-school medicine. We looked at the older surgeons and scoffed at how they ignore the results of randomized, controlled, double-blind studies. Our generation didn't believe in anecdotal science. Anecdotes were for late-night television commercials.

Their "old boys" club consists of curmudgeons and chauvinists. When we went to college, fraternities weren't cool; they were being busted for their cruel hazing rituals. Their generation had its rigid way of climbing ladders and "paying dues." Our generation said, "Forget elbow rubbing and butt kissing, I'm starting my own Internet company."

We were taught that their greed had created a niche for managed care systems. They had started the HMOs that took healthcare money and distributed it to shareholders. Now we had to fix that, too.

We didn't have a reason to respect them. And it was hard to work 130 hours a week for and next to people eager to insult you at any moment. We had all heard that in order to become a surgeon thirty years ago, you had to be ruthless. So, these guys were ruthless? Cheaters? Cunning jerks? And I say "guys" because it was rare to meet a female surgeon over fifty—but we'd change that, too.

Of course, our generation had faults, too. We were just as greedy. Our generation watched "Who Wants to Be a Millionaire?" and "Who Wants to Marry a Millionaire?" Greed was the reason that we don't have loyalty for, or belief in, the businesses we worked in. Our generation looked for the easy dollar. But there was nothing quick and easy about a surgical residency. And our ADHD generation was too shortsighted to imagine a light at the end of a long tunnel.

The conflicts shouldn't have been surprising. Both groups were intelligent, and believed they were always right. Maybe it was surprising that more abuse didn't go on.

*

At midnight a nurse paged me regarding a drop in blood pressure on an ICU patient. The man had had an aortic aneurysm repaired the day before. His blood pressure had remained high after the surgery and his antihypertensive meds had been increased a few hours earlier. Now, suddenly his numbers dropped into the normal range.

I tried to convince myself that his medicines had finally kicked in. His heart rate hadn't changed significantly and his blood pressure had quickly normalized. Great. But something nagged me. I wished I could have communicated with the patient, but he was sedated and intubated.

I knew what was nagging me. Ms. York. The poster-child for the worst-case scenario of a sudden, brief fluctuation in blood pressure. No more fatal heart attacks, please.

I told the nurse to send off stat cardiac labs and to get an EKG.

The labs and EKG confirmed my worries. He had a heart attack. Ms. York's death wasn't futile. I called the junior resident on call and we made sure all the right meds and care were being given and I let him call the attending. No sense in me being the messenger...

The following morning we were supposed to round at seven. Liz actually showed up on time for once and I didn't have my note completed on one of our patients.

"This just won't do. Look at this note; it's not even finished. And you didn't include the fluids from the OR in her 24-hour Is and Os (inputs and outputs)." When she complained, she jutted her head forward and put on a grave look as if everything she was saying was of the utmost importance. I wanted to reach forward and pinch her nose, pinch it hard.

I didn't bother explaining why I was late. No excuse would have been good enough. But for the record, I was taking care of another patient.

"Didn't I say we were meeting at 7?"

I nodded in confirmation.

"Well, I can't have it like this. If this is how it is going to be for the next few weeks, it just won't do. We need to start on time—"

"Just stop," I interrupted. "Fine, I screwed up, but give me this one freebie." I refrained from mentioning how many times she had been late and how insignificant this episode was, but I kept my mouth shut. I was not going to play down on her level.

To my surprise, she actually did shut up. She looked at me with shock and I turned and started walking to our next patient's room.

"So, this won't happen again?" Her voice was timid.

"No." And that ended it. There was no way that wiry headcase could break me, not that close to the end. I didn't want to have to deal with her attitude on top of Rachel dumping me.

Beetle secretly gave me the thumbs up.

News of Ramirez quitting had unsettled the other junior residents. No one expressed concern about Ramirez; instead, they fretted how their workload would increase with another resident gone. And, to guarantee misery, they had fired another junior resident, someone rumored to be a danger to mankind. I asked Corey why they hadn't kept him until the end of the year. He told me that since they fired him early, the year wouldn't count toward finishing residency. He would have to repeat it somewhere else.

Normally I don't swear, but there is no other word for a group of people that would hire someone for a year, cut them loose during the 10th month, and have the whole year not count for anything. Nothing! The only word was Fuckers. The English language is missing out on a polite word for people that do that sort of thing. Corey was wrong. They could stop the clock and the Fuckers just stopped the clock on that poor soul.

These recent events had left a gap at County Hospital that needed to be filled by a resident. Franklin heard it might be him, and he offered his opinion to anyone who would listen: "This is fucking bullshit. No way. No way am I going back there. You have to protect your own, or at least fake like you are trying. I have been completely loyal to this program and they have taken away all my good rotations this year to pull me back there. I am not going back for a fourth time."

I felt sorry for Franklin. They had pulled him off his cake rotation at the beginning of the year to work with Corey, Evan, and me. And, I heard that his fiancée had broken off their engagement a few weeks earlier. Sending him back to County would have been a heaping teaspoon of salt in his wounds.

As per usual, when life gives you crap, look for someone making crap-ade.

One elderly woman obliged and told me a joke about Italians, specifically after confirming my name was Italian.

"Why don't Italians like Jehovah's Witnesses?"

"Why?" I asked.

"They don't like any witnesses."

I asked another woman if she had any other problems besides her breast mass. She complained sometimes black fuzz built up in her belly button. I wanted to praise her for her brilliant deadpan, but she wasn't joking. I smiled at the sincerity of her statement and assured her belly button fuzz is a normal part of life. The abnormal part is wincing while removing it because you're afraid your umbilicus will explode.

It would have been the funniest moment of the day if it weren't for the forty-year-old black man I pre-opped.

He was wearing a patient gown and standing next to the exam table when he asked, "Do I have to take out my piercings for the surgery?"

I had only noticed one ring through his ear. "When you say 'piercings' does that mean you are hiding something I haven't found yet?" I motioned toward his gown.

"Yes, I've got this pierced." He pulled the top of his gown aside to reveal a thick ring through his right nipple. "And I've got this." He lifted his gown. My eyes fell out. Swinging in the breeze was his penis with a metal ring as thick as a pencil through its head. The ring went through his urethral meatus and out the bottom of his penis. Monkeys could have swung from that thing.

"Ahh! Why'd you do that?" The words leaked out before I could squeeze my lips closed.

"You wouldn't believe the sensation. It's great. It's like...I can't even describe it."

"That's okay, you don't have to. I have too much knowledge of anatomy to want to do that to myself." I wondered what it looked like when he peed with the ring out. I imagined a sprinkler system, or Tom Cat full of holes drinking water. You can't believe the sensation...it's like...peeing all over my legs every time I used the bathroom, so warm!

By the time I got home that night, the piercing parlors were closed. Maybe the next day.

Chapter 70

After Grand Rounds, Dr. Organ encouraged all of us to do research. He reminded us for the umpteenth time that he has "tickets reserved for Oslo when we win the Nobel Prize." And for the umpteenth time Brodie almost yelled out, "That's nice, but I'll be in Stockholm to pick up my prize." I hoped that as the year finished Brodie would say it; I was sure the opportunity would arise again.

Then, Dr. Organ called for a private meeting with the residents. He assured next year would be better. There would be more residents to share the work. Rotations would be re-organized. He'd encourage the attendings to do more teaching sessions.

What a timely speech, only a few days after two residents left the program. We all recognized Dr. Organ's transparent attempt to prevent any further departures with vague promises of a better life. But he needed to focus on the junior residents, like Franklin and Barclay. Interns were a dime a dozen, and chiefs weren't a problem because they would do anything to finish their last year. So, at the end of his non-specific assurances and smiles he told the juniors how much he appreciated their hard work and that it wouldn't be forgotten. Then, he told them to look up the word "intern" in the dictionary; he was shocked to see the word "scut" in parentheses. Ha ha ha, very funny.

Their hard work wouldn't be forgotten. He didn't say rewarded or relieved; he said forgotten. Just as the situation with Dr. Irving would be taken care of. That's why Kendra was given the heave-ho. His greasy politician style didn't fool anybody. As we walked out the door Beetle muttered, "Dr. Organ is one of the best spin doctors ever."

*

Liz didn't improve morale either. The stench of laziness emanating from her every action nauseated me. During midday we had a young man come in with probable appendicitis. Liz rehydrated him with IV fluid and gave him antibiotics. A few hours later, we reexamined him. He said his pain had improved some from a few hours ago.

Liz pushed on the right lower quadrant of his abdomen. He winced slightly. She told him that we would probably wait to operate on him, if at all.

As we walked away, I said, "It's better to just get it out if we think he has appendicitis. His white count is still high."

"Well, he might get better just with fluids and antibiotics. Some people do that, you know."

Her opinion contrasted everything Dr. Organ preached. Appendicitis was a clinical diagnosis that requires a surgical cure. Never let the sun set on appendicitis. But those arguments wouldn't appeal to her.

I told her I thought it better to remove it now than the middle of the night.

She gave me her rat grin and accused me of just wanting to take out his appendix.

"Yeah, but only because he needs it out." When in doubt, cut it out. "Let's reexamine him."

She followed me back to him. I laid his bed flat and had him relax. When I palpated his right lower quadrant he tensed up. He involuntarily guarded against my touch, but right before he flexed I felt a small, firm mass.

Liz had him stand up. I watched him wince when he brought his right leg forward. He had appendicitis. His macho act was just that. He couldn't hide appendicitis from the Detective of Bowelsville.

We walked away once again. "He has it," I reaffirmed. "You want to bet a quarter?" Maybe John's tactics would goad her into doing the right thing.

She sighed. "I guess you've convinced me. We'll take it out. I bet the appendix will be laying down into the pelvis and only mildly inflamed."

"Nope, my money is on it being straight up." I think I had the lowest threshold for appendicitis of all the residents. We all listened to Dr. Organ's speeches, but I had a second incentive: A classmate of mine had died of appendicitis in grade school.

A half hour later, the inflamed appendix popped out of the incision I made in the peritoneum like a turtle sticking his head out of his shell. Total time, skin to skin, 27 minutes.

Dr. Iaquinta, you just set the intern land speed record for an appendectomy. What do you have to say?

Well, I'd like to say thanks to all the people with bellyaches. If it weren't for your frequent late-night support of my endeavor, this could have never happened.

Congratulations, Doc. And enjoy your prize: Two hours of

vacation from your busy work schedule. You're extra lucky; your hours off are from eight to ten p.m. next Thursday.

Thanks, Bob.

The next morning my patient ate breakfast without a tinge of pain. Nothing satisfied more than seeing a patient healed. I had actually made a difference in someone's life. If it weren't for me, he wouldn't be eating lousy hospital food.

That is the only reason anyone should become a surgeon: to operate. The selfish secondary gains aren't guaranteed. The public doesn't respect doctors anymore. The money isn't easy to earn and harder to protect from lawsuits. Doctors don't have power; the practice of healthcare is controlled by non-medical administrators. There is no glory. But there is a chance to cut people.

I called Rachel to boast about my speed-appendectomy. She didn't find the achievement monumental. She made no effort whatsoever to contact the local newspapers. And when the conversation was over, I knew that in her mind, our relationship was over. She hung up the phone first.

Chapter 71

I was supposed to remove an abdominal drain from a post-op patient, but when I pulled on it I could feel the tube stretching without the drain moving. The memory of the broken drain left in the abdomen assaulted me. I stopped pulling. Beetle could yank on this one.

Great. Now I was too scared to pull a sticky drain. Next, I wouldn't want to remove any drains. One of these days I'd freeze up at the bedside and they'd wheel me to the loony bin strapped to a dolly.

I called Beetle and told him about the drain. He said he'd rescue me when he got the chance. Meanwhile, I went to unclog someone's feeding tube. I forced Coca-Cola down it until it opened up. If that stuff could take rust off a car, it could dissolve some coagulated tube feed. The old lady expressed her amusement at the novel way of solving her problem until she received the slug of fifty milliliters of Coca-Cola into her belly. Then she puked on me.

Oops. I broke the rule. Never stand within firing range of any orifice.

Beetle paged me as I approached the resident's office. I ducked into the office down the hall and called him.

"Hey, did you get that drain out?" he asked.

"Um, yeah. Can you get up here, right now?" I blurted.

"What's going on?'"

"I got that drain out, but now he is spurting blood from the drain hole!"

"Holy cats! I thought you were going to have me do it."

"I didn't want to waste time, hurry up here, I have the nurse holding pressure."

"I'll be right..."

I hung up on him and giggled.

I ran out into the hallway. He raced out of the resident's office like a running back trying to get the last yard on fourth down. He almost plowed me over as he turned the corner. I burst into laughter.

"Oh man, you are dead. You totally had me going."

"Sorry, that was cruel, but so darn funny." I snickered. There was so much fun to be had!

Karma got me back for him. Karma came in the form of a wound-care nurse named Natalie. She asked me to watch her debride a man's pressure ulcer. I suggested I wasn't the right person for the task, but she insisted to have me oversee her scrape off some dead tissue from some guy's sacral decubitus ulcer (an ulcer at the base of the spine just above the buttocks).

When I got there she handed me a mask. "Wear this and only breathe through your mouth. The nurses haven't been taking care of him because he smells so bad."

The odor knocked me backward. I had memories of finding a dead raccoon behind the barn one July. That raccoon smelled like flowers compared to this guy.

When we rolled him onto his side, a jetstream of stench pummeled us. I gagged silently.

He had a circle of wrinkled, dead skin the size of a salad plate just above his butt on his lower back. I saw a wave ripple underneath it as we moved him.

Why am I here?

Natalie answered the question for me. To cut people.

She held up the scalpel for a second—just to make sure I was watching. She poked the center of the ulcer with her scalpel. The skin fell apart like wet tissue paper, and a thick yellow bisque of pus flowed from the wound. She peeled away the loosely hanging flesh that had covered the abscess cavity, and then she scraped the mucous webs out of the wound. I grabbed the wall suction catheter and stuck it into the wound. It made this repulsive slurping noise and the tubing filled with thick yellow pus. I had that nasty taste in the back of my mouth that meant there was a high likelihood that I would blow chunks imminently.

I lurched out of the room. But, the stench stuck in my nose. I couldn't escape it. Then I realized I didn't know what should be done for the patient. He had a big hole in his back. Hanging him up by his arms and spraying his lower back with a fire hose was my best idea. So, I paged Beetle.

"Beetle, you have to come see this wound. I'm not sure how to treat it."

"What are you doing seeing a wound?"

"I don't know. The wound care nurse asked me to help her. But it's so big and nasty that it freaks me out. You have to see it. And when you come, wear a mask and don't breathe through your nose."

"Right, this is another one of your jokes. I am not falling for it."

"No, really, this guy has a lake of pus. You have to see it. It's a lake of pus. It's the most disgusting thing I've ever seen. I am thanking God at this very moment that I am not staying in General Surgery. This is the sacral decube that will make you want to go into anesthesiology."

"Are you lying?" I heard a glimmer of hope in his voice. Maybe this wound would change his life.

"No, get up here and see this. This isn't the boy crying wolf."

Beetle showed up, and, he wrinkled his nose. After a cursory examination he admitted that the wound was indeed reason not to pursue a career in General Surgery. Then to make things grosser, he asked the wound care nurse if maggots would be any help.

Seriously. The guy was too sick to go to the OR. But maggots could debride the wound by eating all the dead tissue. Talk about a non-stop ticket to Vomitville.

Nobody is cut out for this.

*

Liz rarely interacted with me after I stopped her from reprimanding me. So she started taking all her aggressions out on Beetle.

First of all, she made Beetle scrub in to assist her with an above-the-knee amputation, clearly an intern-level case. He grumbled about being on call, but Liz didn't relent. Instead she had me take his pager. Good thing I was a white cloud; not a single page came in.

After that case, Liz decided that we would take on another team's patient so that they could go home. I would have given her credit for the magnanimous gesture, but she let them know she was their savior a little too loudly. But what did they care? They got to go home.

Our new patient was an 11-year-old with ruptured appendicitis. She needed an exploratory laparotomy.

And I got to do it.

I hadn't heard of any of the other interns getting to do an ex-lap, but there I was cutting through a young girl's abdomen to get to the bowel. I couldn't slice her open with the speed that Corey did, but I still did the cut in one smooth motion.

She had a generous layer of subcutaneous fat. No shortage of plump eleven-year-olds these days. I effortlessly dissected through it down to the peritoneum. Liz commented on my clean, dry dissection.

We found a ruptured appendix and other "intraloop" abscesses. We tried to untangle her inflamed bowel. She had pockets of pus everywhere, even around her ovaries and tubes.

Dr. Kudrow came in to look over my shoulder. "Irrigate her out with forty liters of saline; it's the only chance she has to remain fertile."

After we flushed her out, Liz let me close the abdomen. I was surprised Dr. Kudrow hadn't said anything about me doing the case, or warned me about stitching the drain in. Somehow, he must have developed trust in me. That was my moment to prove him wrong and yank the girl's spleen out with my hand and eat it like an apple.

Beetle should have done the case, but Liz had some sort of point to prove that night. I think she overheard him referring to her by one of her many nicknames. But which one? The Queen. The Bitch. The Little Princess. The Heiress. That Fuckin' Liz. The Psychopath. Idiot. The Devil. The Fuckin' Bitch. Queenie.

At 2 a.m. Beetle paged me.

"Hello," I answered groggily.

"We have to take a paraplegic woman to the OR to drain some butt pus, but Liz wants me to do it."

My sleepy self wanted to demand why he bothered calling me if I wasn't doing the case, but I held back. There had to be a reason. "What do you need me to do?"

"I need you to come down here and provide emotional support and comic relief. She is going to kill me—if I don't kill her."

So, I went down, made bad jokes, wrote the orders, and drifted back upstairs to sleep for a couple hours. You didn't need to know Beetle long to want to grant him such a favor.

I started putting the cookies and Coca-Cola from our conference box lunches in Beetle's desk drawer. I also gave him the days off when only one of us had to come in. It wasn't pure generosity; I had schemed up a plan to finish the year two days early. If he covered rounding for me the last weekend then I'd be done with internship on a Friday night. I worried that leaving early might weaken this narrative, but concluded that I'd rather the Reader suffer than myself.

Chapter 72

I had a two-day "vacation" from the hospital to take Step 3 of the Boards. Taking a test eight hours a day for two days was a break from getting up at 5:00 to work an unpredictable number of hours. The concept seemed so relaxing that I found it hard to be stressed out over another major exam.

But working with Liz after a two-day hiatus was like returning to Wisconsin in January after a week in Key West; I hadn't realized how acclimated I had become to her coldness.

I found Beetle in the resident's room talking on the phone. I could tell by the way he moaned "yes" into the receiver that he was talking to the She-Devil. He groaned a final yes and then hung up the phone.

"Ahhh!" He repeatedly slammed the phone into its cradle. "Could I"—slam—"possibly"—slam—"hate someone"—slam—"more than I..."—slam—

"Um, no?" I guessed.

While I took the test, Liz pushed Beetle to the brink. I didn't ask what happened; I just shouted with glee when Beetle told me he sent off applications to anesthesia programs.

We danced our way to the Pediatric floor. I offered to swipe him an ice cream to celebrate his new future. En route, we found ourselves alone in the elevator with the wound care nurse.

"I wonder if you could help me again," she began. She had freckles and a cute smile, but I knew she worked for the dark side.

I pleaded for her to accost some other resident. I even offered to bribe her with ice cream.

"I'm just kidding. You don't have to help. He died yesterday."

I made the sign of the cross and silently thanked God.

Cripes, look how callous I'd become.

Chapter 73

Rachel's last visit would best be described as "suspension of disbelief." Neither of us said or did anything that hinted June was just around the corner. We simply enjoyed each other.

Or maybe, we were both really good at not saying anything. I knew if the weekend were good enough, she might just change her mind about the break-up. And I also knew that discussing it wouldn't win her over, nor would flowers, but I tried a hefty dose of the latter just in case I was wrong.

The only thing I thought would change her heart was that if she felt the way I did when we were together. The rest of the world didn't exist. A hike in the Berkeley hills, sushi, a movie, we were both on a vacation soaking up every moment.

Maybe it was just her being polite to me, but I think she was savoring every last moment of our relationship, too. By the end of the weekend my attempt to subtly convince her to defer the June first deadline had worked its magic on me. There was no way she could call it off. If a couple like us could separate just because of distance, what hope did the rest of the world have?

But as soon as I left her at the airport a nagging feeling crept into my brain. What if she really does it? I could have asked at the very end of the trip. A quick "Are we still off for June first?" But I didn't, because I was afraid.

When I went to bed that night, the pillow smelled like her shampoo. I already missed her.

Chapter 74

Monday didn't care that I had the weekend off, and I had call that night. We started the evening by admitting a crazy woman with gangrenous hemorrhoids. I understand that crazy is an oft used adjective that usually does not mean truly crazy. But Mrs. Christian was crazy. She had been discharged from the Medicine service a few days before, and on her way out of the hospital she had dialed the suicide hotline from the lobby and said that not only was she suicidal but her husband was trying to kill her.

Psychiatry had seen her and concluded that she had personality problems, but they couldn't diagnose her for a true psychiatric illness. I told the psychiatrist that if the patient wasn't ill, maybe we should bring in her husband and evaluate him. After all, you'd have to be somewhat insane to try to kill a suicidal person.

Not that a psych diagnosis would have saved us from treating her giant hemorrhoids. And now that shrink declared her "normal-ish," we could consent her for surgery.

She didn't want to be all the way asleep for the surgery so we used spinal anesthesia to paralyze her from the hips down. Spinal anesthetic leaves the patient unable to urinate. We told her that she would need a Foley catheter until the anesthetic wore off. She consented.

At the end of the case I wrote the usual orders. But I also added "the patient will require much patience and finesse on the part of the nursing staff."

At 2:30 a.m. I received the first page. Mrs. Christian claimed the nurses were torturing her because they wouldn't remove the Foley catheter. I told them that she knew she needed it and I wasn't going to consent its removal.

At 3 a.m. they paged again. "Mrs. Christian is trying to get ahold of her lawyer. She says she's being tortured. She yanked out the Foley herself, with the balloon up."

I could hear her screaming in the background, "Is that the doctor, I want to talk to him, I shouldn't be here." The nurse told her no. I got the name of the nurse and wrote her a letter of commendation.

At 3:15 the nurse paged to tell me that Mrs. Christian had yanked out her IV. She didn't want any medications. I told the nurse to explain that she wouldn't get the IV antibiotics she needed to prevent infection. "If she doesn't want it reinserted, just document it. Did you read my orders? She needs to be handled with finesse. I can't come down there and magically cure her psychosis."

At 3:30 a.m. she paged again. She wanted the Foley reinserted because she couldn't pee. The nurses wanted to restrain her because she was chasing them down the hallway. "Fine, do whatever you want, but don't call me again. There is nothing else I can do."

And they didn't call again.

The next morning Beetle called Psych to have her re-evaluated. They weren't interested. But Beetle was on his toes. "But, sir, she was telling the governor to get out of her room this morning."

I raised my eyebrows skeptically. Beetle hung up. "What was that about?"

"Just a little embellishment so they come see her."

Psych called our bluff. They remained unimpressed by her anxiety and had no new recommendations. So much for taking her away in one of those little padded trucks.

When I signed her out to Evan that evening, he seemed as disinterested in her lunacy as everyone else. He hoped she'd be going home. But he did ask, "What did gangrenous hemorrhoids look like?"

"It looked like someone had turned a baby inside out and stuck it to her butt."

*

I found out from an intern who returned from burn rotation that both the little girl and the man with over 90% burns were still alive. Both were beating the odds.

I also found out that the burn service had admitted twelve other people with greater than 90% burns in the first ten days after I left. See, I am a white cloud.

Chapter 75

When I returned there was a note on the computer from Evan. It read "Sorry. Still here. Talk to me about it." And there was an arrow pointing to "Mrs. Christian."

Shoot. The deal I made with her the day before was that if she had a bowel movement she could go home.

When I walked into her room, she returned my greeting with, "Where were you? That doctor you had covering while you were gone took a half hour to respond to my call yesterday. And then I found out he was here in the hospital. I had pain with my bowel movement. It was improper of him to not give me Demerol for my pain." A tear came to her eye. "Where were you? Did you have a good time golfing? He might be your friend and all, but you shouldn't have people like that cover for you."

She was a skinny woman. All the crazy people were. Liz was scrawny, too. Neck muscles and veins sticking out all over the place. It must have taken a lot of energy to be insane; they burned off all those calories with crazy thoughts. I reminded myself that I was a caring doctor. Sticks and stones may break my bones but words would never hurt me.

"I understand you were in pain. However, none of the medicines we give you are going to take away all the pain. I agree with the other doctor's decision not to give you intravenous narcotics every time you pass your bowels. The Sitz baths should help the surgical site relax; have you been taking them?"

"No, I just felt like lying in bed yesterday."

"Well, you are supposed to be doing those three times a day. They will help ease the pain. You did prove to us yesterday that you could have a bowel movement. The nursing chart reports that you had four of them. From my standpoint you are still fit to go home."

"Well, if I am going to go home I need a prescription for all of my medicines."

That's it? Just some prescriptions? I was getting off easy.

But, I was paged an hour later. More complaints.

"You said you were going to give me the medicines I had. I need Fiorinal with codeine, Vicodin, and Tylenol with codeine. Then I want some of that Ativan that the doctor gave me yesterday."

She had asked for a handbasket of narcotics and a Tylenol overdose. She didn't know that the computer had flashed "Warning. Patient has drug-seeking behavior" when I had checked out her medication history.

"Fiorinal is a medication for migraines. You need to have that refilled by the doctor who treats you for those. And, I will only prescribe the Vicodin or the Tylenol with codeine. If I gave you both you would risk overdosing on Tylenol. As for the Ativan, I did not write for you to have it. It is very good at reducing anxiety, but the psychiatrist does not recommend any medication for you."

"Was the psychiatrist the gray-haired guy who came in here for forty seconds yesterday morning and told me he liked the classical music I was listening to?"

"I'm not sure." Stinking psychiatrist—if he spent a whole forty seconds with her he could have made a diagnosis.

"Is there any sleeping medicine that you can give me? How about Seconal?"

No way. I negotiated her down to a lower-potency sleeping medicine. Everything was agreed upon. Almost.

"But Doctor, I didn't have a bowel movement today. It has been almost 14 hours."

According to the nurse she had had one late the night before. "You proved to us that you have a patent conduit. What is going in is coming out, and I see no reason why that should have changed in the last 12 hours."

"Are you sure? I don't want to come right back here because I don't have a bowel movement."

BELIEVE ME, I DON'T WANT YOU TO EITHER. I assured her that she'd have future bowel movements. Loose ones, to prevent straining and stressing the operative site.

She accused me of just trying to get her out of my hair.

You are absolutely right. "No, it is not that. But you are ready to go. I want you to understand that you are running the normal course and what to expect. And, I wasn't golfing yesterday evening; I do get to go home now and then."

"Well, what were you doing?"

"Catching up on my sleep. I was up all night the night before." No thanks to you.

And I escaped. The medicine residents warned me that it would be a struggle to discharge her. This wasn't a struggle; it was an all-out battle.

Not a half hour later, the nurse told me that the patient didn't think she could go because she was sure she parked her car in a garage that was locked over the weekend. I told the nurse if security couldn't open the gates I would blast them open for her.

I went back to the floor a few hours later and tiptoed up to Mrs. Christian's door. I peeked an eye around it. A nurse came up behind me and called my name. I jumped forward. The bed was empty!

"Doctor, she left an hour ago."

"I'm free!" I waved my arms in the air.

*

Beetle and I snuck outside to throw my Frisbee around. I looked up at the ugly hospital and I saw the curtain move in chief's call room. "Liz just pulled her curtain shut."

"She's probably lounging in bed as usual. She's always up there. I hate it. Whenever she hears me go into my room I get a page a minute later and she gives me some stupid task to do."

"She's done that to me, but now I tiptoe in and close the door silently."

"I brought some WD-40 in because my door would squeak," Beetle admitted.

The brilliance of a mechanic.

A page interrupted our game. I thought it was going to be Liz, but it was a number I had never seen before. I went in to the surgery clinic to make my call.

"Hello, Doctor. It's me, Mrs. Christian. I needed to talk to you. I haven't had a bowel movement yet."

"How did you get my pager number?"

"I saw it on the chart. I'm sure you won't make that mistake ever again."

Arrgh. "No, the proper way to get a hold of me is through the surgery advice answering service. But, now that we are talking, how are you doing?"

"I haven't gone to the bathroom all day."

"You just went last night. You had four bowel movements yesterday; I would be surprised if you had any bowel movement today." I picked up a pencil and started doodling on my census sheet.

"But I am really scared. What if I have a blockage and nothing can get out?"

"We both know that isn't true. You had a bowel movement last night. There is no reason for it to block off overnight."

"But I ate All Bran, and a banana, I had a heaping teaspoon of Metamucil with water and some fortified orange juice—I need the extra vitamins, you know—and some Colace. I was just about to start sipping that fruity solution. Should I come in?"

"No, but if you don't have one by Tuesday afternoon you can come to our clinic. I doubt that we would find anything new, but this gives us a plan of attack." By now I had a figure hanging from a noose sketched on my paper. Cleaner than burning to death.

"Okay."

"And remember, don't take the sorbitol, the fruity stuff, unless you go more than another day without a bowel movement." What she really needed was a hobby. If she spent her time doodling she wouldn't obsess about her bowel movements all day long.

When I went upstairs, Liz yelled at me for not checking a lab for her. My punishment was that I couldn't round on our ICU patients anymore. Beetle would have to do it all alone.

When I told Beetle, he christened her "The Almighty Bitch." Only an Almighty Bitch, not a regular Bitch, would punish him by making me do less work.

*

I tried to avoid it, but I could not escape the fact that it was June first. When I got home I made the call. I didn't want to, but I had to know.

"It's June first" I stated.

"Yes," she confirmed.

"Does that mean...?"

"Yes."

"Can we move it to August first, or September?"

307

"Nope, you said June."

Drats. It was just like me to have my life so scheduled that we would break up on the day I had chosen, albeit jokingly. The whole thing seemed so silly that I had a hard time feeling sad, for a couple of minutes.

Chapter 76

The next morning I did all my usual pre-rounding on the ICU players, but I put the notes in my pocket instead of leaving them in the chart. Then, when Beetle showed up, I told him to say that he didn't pre-round because it was not a junior resident's responsibility to pre-round.

We waited the usual ten minutes for Liz to come marching in.

Beetle and I had developed a Pavlovian response to the quick clacking of Liz's shoes approaching from down the hall. Beetle said, "Here come the little hooves," and we would grimace and cringe in fear. Sometimes, if we leaned forward far enough over the nurse's desks, we were obscured from her by the milieu of meandering nurses.

As usual, Liz busted us trying to hide from her.

Liz asked, "So, how is everyone doing?"

Normally I wouldn't have been able to keep a straight face to pull this off, but if Mrs. Christian's lunacy taught me one thing, it was how to suppress a grin. "I don't know. I didn't bother coming early since I lost note-writing privileges."

She turned to Beetle. He stammered, "I just thought you were kidding. When we left last night you didn't say anything. Pre-rounding is the intern's job."

She looked back at me. I shrugged. She looked at Beetle. He just looked her back in the eye. Beetle sat there like the Cincinnati Kid, not a facial twitch.

She grinned and shook her head, like she was dealing with idiots. "Well, all right. Let's go."

Disappointment? Where's the tirade? You were supposed to get all worked up.

"I'm just kidding. Here are the notes."

"I was only five minutes late, that's not late enough to deserve pranks. I'm sure I broke the speed limit getting here."

She obviously didn't know me well. If I didn't play pranks, I wouldn't have anything to play...we all know it's not the piano.

*

Later that morning, Mrs. Christian paged again. I didn't want to call her, but I reasoned that if I didn't, she would come in.

"Hello, Doctor, sorry to bother you but I wanted to let you know what was going on."

"What is going on?"

"Yesterday morning I was scared that I wasn't going to have a bowel movement. I had bran for breakfast, my Metamucil, then, I took some of the Colace and ate some fruit. But nothing, so I started drinking that fruity solution. I ended up sipping it here and there and I drank the whole bottle over a few hours."

I had prescribed a 300 ml bottle. A single dose is 15 ml. That usually sent the most constipated ass trotting to the bathroom. The directions say to wait six hours between doses.

She continued, "But then I just wouldn't stop going to the bathroom. I couldn't even leave the toilet. At first, I was having normal formed stools, but then they became diarrhea. Some would even leak out whenever I'd walk. I feared that the surgery made me incontinent. I would have been the world's worst dance partner."

Finally, someone who is a worse dance partner than me. "Oh, that's disgusting." I imagined her butt looking like an exploded cigar and her twirling around like a ballerina spraying diarrhea everywhere. "Did you use the Sitz baths?"

"Yes, but when I sat down more stool would come out of me. I just couldn't stop it."

Pooping in the tub is not cool.

"Mrs. Christian, we need to get you on a normal bowel regimen. Right now you are riding the teeter-totter all the way up and slamming into the ground. You need balance. First of all, no more sorbitol."

"I ran out." She finished a week's worth in one day.

Good. Maybe that alone would break this cycle. I recited to her what I hypothesized would be a good bowel regimen.

At the end of all her okays she asked, "Do you think I'll have a bowel movement again?"

AHHHHH! Normally I don't make any guarantees, as there are none. But in this case, I guaranteed she'd have a bowel movement again, I didn't tack on the disclaimer "unless you die first." Then I tried to give myself some leeway by telling her that her system was so empty it'd be a few days.

She finally hung up. The poor woman obsessed about her bowel movements so much that she couldn't even function, couldn't even leave the house. But then I couldn't stop imagining her running through her house, dripping diarrhea as she tried to make it to the bathroom. Sharing poop stories is just one of the many responsibilities of having a Y chromosome. I immediately paged Beetle and told him about the "World's Worst Dance Partner."

That evening Dhara and I went out to a Vietnamese restaurant. I hadn't seen her in a month. I think every time we met we spent the first half of the visit sharing horrible stories. Hers were usually worse; as an Ob-Gyn resident, it meant half her bad stories included babies. None of mine had a dead baby multiplier. And she didn't have a Rachel equivalent, so many of her stories she hadn't discussed with anyone else.

She told me about her previous night call. She had to do a C-section on one patient and had another six in labor, all with potentially complicated deliveries, plus other patients. The nurses hadn't paged her when two of her patient's blood pressures skyrocketed. She discovered the changes in vital signs fortuitously while rounding between cases. She said when she finished call she was just thankful that none of her patients had died.

I realized that a single doctor could be sued for simultaneous events. All six of the patients in labor had specific orders that she was to be called if the blood pressure exceeded the written parameters. While she performed a C-section, the other two patients or their unborn babies could have suffered complications from the high BP. Both could have sued, simply because the nursing staff wasn't doing their job. Why would anyone want to be a doctor?

I asked Dhara if she told the nurses about the missed calls. She hadn't. I told her the story about Mr. Leigh and his near overdose of narcotics. I had tried to tell the nurse what was wrong, but was met with apathy, so I transferred the patient. Dhara felt that in her case it was safer not to create any enemies with the nursing staff. If anyone could have done things politely, it was Dhara. I had the sense she didn't stick up for herself and the patients the way she should. For herself, in general.

When I got home, Rachel called. I told her that I hung out with Dhara for a few hours. "How was your date?" she asked.

"I wouldn't call it a date. There was no hand-holding or smooches." I started to pace a hole in the carpet. Her line of questioning was not fair.

"It wasn't a romantic dinner?"

"No. Somehow she made no attempt to throw herself at me once I revealed you dumped me. And, you can't do that. You can't break up with me and then harass me about having dinner with a woman."

"Just because we aren't together doesn't mean I still don't like you."

I offered to take her back. But she declined. She couldn't "do a long-distance relationship."

We were at an impasse. But she couldn't tease me about Dhara. Hadn't she read the Rule Book? She had broken up with me; therefore, she had forfeited her harassing rights. It was in the chapter right after calling "uno" after the second to last straw.

Chapter 77

The next afternoon, after I finished operating, I found a message from Mrs. Christian waiting for me. My fascination with the sick and twisted won out, I called her back.

Zero progress. "You know how I told you about how runny my stool was Monday night? I dirtied every towel in the house that day. It was horrible. The towels are just disgusting. But when I lifted that bag of towels I had a pain shoot down to my tailbone. I think I might be blocked up."

"I don't think so, Mrs. Christian." I grabbed my pen and started sketching.

"I am afraid that I have a big tumor blocking things up. It's probably hanging off my uterus."

I assured her that her bowels, uterus, and CT scan were all normal. Everything was normal except her bowel regimen and her brain. By the time I convinced her that she didn't need any more scans, I had drawn a little man kneeling with his head under a guillotine.

"Maybe I just feel sorry for myself. I just want to move my bowels."

"Mrs. Christian, you seem really upset. Would you be interested in talking to someone about your concerns? Someone who can spend more time with you and discuss your worries?"

"Ha! I've been seeing the same psychiatrist for the last 25 years."

Well he needs his license revoked. "Okay, it's just that I am not going to be doing General Surgery here after the next two weeks and I don't think that your problem is a surgical issue."

"Where are you going? Are you going into private practice?"

She was missing the point.

She continued. "So you want this to be our last conversation? You don't want some kooky old lady calling you up?"

"Well…" I hesitated; no sense lying. "Ideally yes, but I don't want to leave you without you feeling that you have adequate follow-up."

I changed my position on suing on the grounds of suffering. I know I said life was full of anguish. But if people get to sue for suffering, then I wanted to sue my patients! Did they know how much anguish they put me through? Keeping me up all night worrying about them, trying to treat them, trying to keep their hearts beating, trying to make them accept their bowel function, making me deal with their psychiatric illnesses. I bet I've suffered more than most of them—well, the live ones.

Chapter 78

When I woke up that morning I found my pager vibrating its way across the carpet. I scrolled through the numerous pages. The first number was evidence that a nurse had paged me instead of the on-call intern. The next four numbers however, were the same number, Mrs. Christian's. 9:40 p.m. 11:46 p.m. 2:15 a.m. 5:07 a.m.

My first thought was *Fatal Attraction*. I'd come home one night and find a rabbit on the stove and Mrs. Christian on my toilet.

6:20 a.m.: another page.

6:46 a.m.: another page.

6:54 a.m.: another page.

By the third page, Liz and Beetle stopped teasing that I had already found a new girlfriend and started offering advice. Get a new pager. Go to the attending. Wait two weeks.

7:16 a.m.: another page.

I wasn't going to call back until I could ensure it would be my last time.

9:03 a.m.: A floor nurse pages me. "Doctor, a Mrs. Christian keeps calling here asking for you. She is crying that she needs to talk to you."

"Thank you, but tell her the proper way to get ahold of me is through the advice line. She has the number."

9:27 a.m.: another page.

I found the attending that I did her case with and he offered to see her in his clinic four days from then. "From now on," he said, "her only surgical care is through me. Have the clinic call her and tell her that."

I went the rest of the day without another page. But still put in a request for a new pager.

Beetle paged me that evening.

"Guess who's down here in the ER?"

"Who?"

"Your buddy, Mrs. Christian."

"NO!"

"Yeah. I just saw her on a gurney on her way to x-ray."

"Tell the ER doctors her history. Don't let them waste time

working her up. And, no matter what, don't admit her. Don't even accept a consult from them. Tell them she is Dr. Hunt's private patient and that she has an appointment on Monday."

"Don't worry. I'll stay far away."

Beetle did sneak down and look at her x-ray. She had a bunch of stool in her rectum, undoubtedly the fiber she had stuffed herself with. A paradoxical constipation can result from eating too much fiber without drinking enough water.

Late at night, Beetle and I sometimes treated ourselves to ice cream from the pediatrics floor or Cup-of-Soup from the recovery room. After sleep rounds, Beetle asked if I had had a snack yet.

"No, they're all out of soup."

He immediately broke into a new version of the Air Supply song. "I'm all out of soup, I'm so lost without soup." Beetle confessed that he was a singing telegram for part of his late college career.

While we futilely searched for soup, Beetle told me everything was "in place" for him to leave the program and go into the anesthesia program.

"What is the number one factor that is holding you back?"

"I like some of it. If you take away the general malaise and melancholy of this place, operating is fun. Plus, I think I'd be good at it. If I make it through this, I have a job waiting for me."

"What are you going to do?"

"I don't know. I think I'm going to get some ice cream." I followed him upstairs to raid the sick kids' refrigerator.

I got one page that night at 4:56 a.m. Mrs. Christian. The ER mustn't have wanted her.

*

That evening I went to rent a movie and coincidentally bumped into Dhara. We decided to watch a movie at my place.

Rachel called during the movie. I debated whether or not to tell her that Dhara was over. I didn't want to upset her, but decided it would be deceitful not to tell her. So, I told Rachel that we were watching a movie. Rachel said "Okay" and hung up on me.

Ouch.

I called Rachel back after Dhara left. She hardly gave me a chance

316

to explain that I bumped into Dhara in the store and this hadn't been a date. She continued to be irritated.

I finally got sick of it.

"Stop teasing me about her. She is one of the only friends I have out here and you try to make me feel guilty every time I hang out with her. We only see each other once every three or four weeks."

"Do you think you could date her?"

"I don't know. When I am with her I don't find myself wishing we were dating. When she leaves at the end of the evening I don't find myself wanting to kiss her goodbye."

"What about in the future?"

"I can't predict the future."

"I just get insecure when you hang out with her."

"But why her more than any other girl I ever hung out with?"

"I don't know, maybe because she's your friend, and you usually date people you've been friends with first."

I told her she was being unfair. She knew I had more women friends than men. And she hung out with guys all the time, even tricked them into giving her and her roommate massages.

"I know, but I'm worried."

"About what?" *That you made a mistake?*

"I don't know what I want. I'm afraid of the day that you call me and say you've started dating someone else."

"Then why did you break up with me?"

"I don't know. It just seemed logical."

"One of these days one of us is going to start dating someone else."

"I know." She started crying. "But I can't imagine how much it will hurt."

"Rachel, I'm not looking for someone to date right now. I don't even feel like we've broken up yet." *Why am I consoling you when you dumped me? That's against the rules!*

"I know, I feel like that, too. Nothing bad came between us; we're just too far apart. I am just not ready for this. I love you."

"I love you, too." *If you really love me, then date me anyway. I'll*

317

have more time to travel next year, so will you. I didn't tell her my thoughts, because if our weekend together didn't convince her, how could a couple of sentences?

*

I called my friend Tyler, the organic chemist, to talk to him about it. He said the same thing Corey had said: I was an idiot. But he also said, "I think it is one of the biggest mistakes of our generation; we blow off love for our careers. When you find someone great you have to keep her. What good is it to be a great doctor fifteen years from now if you have no one to share it with? Is she great?" he asked.

"Yeah. She is a combination of intelligence and humor, and she likes to do things. It's like Dungeons & Dragons. The Elf has 16 points for speed but only 4 for strength. The Wizard has 17 points for magic but only 8 for speed. . ."

"So, she's got an 18 for charisma."

"She's got high numbers across the board."

"Then you shouldn't break up. I know how picky you are. People like that don't just come along every day. If it weren't for my wife pointing me in the right direction, I wouldn't be here. Sure, I would have done things differently. I probably would have traveled more, and maybe never stopped. I'd probably be some bum by now, maybe even served time. But she added direction in my life."

I started cutting my bagel in half. I had been on a streak of eating bagel sandwiches (lettuce, tomato, sliced meat du jour) when I got home at night. It was probably the twentieth in a row. "But, you two had time to spend together. We didn't have much time before we started long distance. It is hard to know how much we like being together if we never are."

"But, you already know you love each other. The rest you can work out. You aren't going to find the ideal person where neither of you has to struggle. Almost any two people could get together and make it work; they just have to put forth the effort."

I knew that was true; there was, after all, a long history of successful arranged marriages. But I didn't want to have to struggle too much. Wasn't that what residency was for?

We went on to define love, the steps to a 100% successful relationship, and then we figured out who really murdered JFK. But I won't bore you with those things.

Chapter 79

Beetle and I went to the cafeteria for lunch. He asked for the minestrone, but they didn't have any left.

"Arrg, no more soup!" he exclaimed.

Doing the best I could with my less than melodious voice, I sang, "I'm all out of soup, I'm so lost without soup."

He couldn't tell if I was mocking him or just a really lousy singer.

So I bought him lunch.

But he ultimately paid. Mrs. Christian showed up to his clinic. She tried to convince him that she hadn't had a bowel movement in weeks because of an obstructing tumor. She insisted she wasn't getting the care she needed. And she was right; she needed a psychiatrist.

Beetle tried to tell her that he knew the truth but she wouldn't hear of it. Then he told her that she had eaten too much fiber and that it constipated her. To which she replied, "Don't tell me about fiber. I know the up, down, left, right about fiber. I have been eating this much fiber for years."

Apparently she didn't know the in and out about fiber. Ba-da-bump.

*

I thought Rachel and I could work out. I had been thinking and rethinking what I thought was our only option. I was convinced she could rotate at a hospital near me for her fourth year. Our medical school allowed a number of away rotations. If she did, then we'd only have to make it one more year before we could spend a significant amount of time together. It was the only chance we had.

I called her immediately. "Have you thought about rotating out here your fourth year?"

"I thought about it. What do you want?"

This time I didn't screw it up. I didn't hesitate. I knew what I wanted. "I think we should keep dating, and then next year you could spend most of the year out here."

"I might come out, but I still think we need to be apart this year. I can't do this long-distance relationship. I need someone to hang out with. Someone I can spend time with at least a few times a week."

It felt like she had reached through mouthpiece, down my throat, and shoved a tennis ball down my esophagus. "Oh."

She continued, "It's not that I want to date anyone else, and if I did, it would have to be someone I thought I was going to marry. But I can't continue dating you long distance."

Her voice was too determined for any rebuttal. This was going to hurt worse than the usual post-relationship blues where I was convinced I'd lost the best thing in the universe. That's exactly what it was, but this time it wouldn't be a teenage over-exaggeration.

Chapter 80

This was part of the email my friend, Lisa, sent me:

> How is your skill at public speaking lately? (This was where my hands started sweating.) Jimmy and I are having two Bible passages (yawn) and one sonnet by Shakespeare (my favorite) read at our wedding. We would be honored if you would read the sonnet for us. (By now my posture was a perfect letter C.) It will take some practice, and it is also very meaningful to me so you can't mumble it…mumbler. The fringe benefit to this task is that you get to come to the rehearsal dinner, which is at this killer Italian restaurant.

I guessed word of my triumphant aortic balloon pump presentation finally made it to Southern California. But reading a sonnet at a wedding in front of people seemed a lot closer to a piano recital than talking to a bunch of half-asleep doctors at seven in the morning.

Chapter 81

Liz was gone in spirit, and almost physically. She spent her days preparing for life after graduation. Beetle and I found her to be a much better chief in absentia. This way she wouldn't poison our minds with her crazy treatment plans. My favorite quote of hers will stick with me forever. She said, "I know the other surgeons don't do it this way, and the literature doesn't support it, but this is how I like to do it." That's priceless.

After early afternoon rounds, she left us to finish the cases and floor work. Liz had convinced the attending to let her go "pick up someone from the airport."

Beetle and I knew she went shopping with her family and then out to eat. I think she told us her hooky plans just so she could rub it in. I hated that gloating rat grin.

At 10:30 p.m. Liz got me out of bed to ask how our patients were doing. I curtly told her everyone had died and asked that she let me go back to sleep.

The next evening was the surgery department dinner. It was the first time most of the faculty had seen me in something besides scrubs. I went overboard with a tuxedo, but if you own one you have to make up reasons to wear it.

Dr. Organ said, "Iaquinta, you can't come to next year's party unless you make a sudden change of plans."

I laughed in his face.

Chapter 82

My last night on call. Had they known, I'm sure they would have trickled patients in all night long. But after operating for eleven hours, things quieted down. I expected something major, an event or a realization. A few easy calls, but nothing to sweat.

Maybe nothing happened because they knew they had missed their chance. I wouldn't break on the last call. Nobody breaks on the last call. No, they were all too busy scheming how they would torture the new interns the following week.

*

My plot worked. I got the last weekend off, which meant Friday was my last day.

I woke up at 4:30 a.m. to pre-round. Never again would I round that early. At 5 a.m., a nurse told me that I looked "buoyant."

Then, a fortuitous chain of events—including one attending going to a meeting, another vacationing, and another canceling a major case—meant we had little to do. Beetle and I went for cereal rounds. This meant raiding the pediatric floor for Rice Krispies. Those stories about starving interns stealing food off the trays of sleeping patients are true...but only from patients with weaker grips than us.

I had Beetle autograph the back of my certificate of completion. I promised him that when he became famous I would hang it backward in its frame so everyone could see I had worked under him.

Liz ran errands for three hours and returned in the evening. At our parting she said to me, "You did a good job. I know I was hard on you these last two months." She reached up and gave me a hug. My insides twisted, nearly obstructing my bowels. But after they realized an obstruction would keep me in the hospital, they straightened out.

I was too excited to run out the door to care what Liz said. I didn't waste time telling her off. I was on my way...home, sweet home.

None of my attendings acknowledged my leaving. Not a single "thank you" or "good luck." The nurses didn't stick their heads out the windows and blow trumpets and kisses. Each intern had his or her own victory. The clock didn't stop for any of us, and only me and my mom cared.

Day 364 and on. . .

I made it, and without buying a palm pilot. And I have more hair on my head than I thought I would have. I thought I'd look like Corey.

Only by comparing the last day to the first could I realize the progression. I had done more than run errands. They had introduced me to the operating room. On my last day, I noticed how comfortably I manipulated the tissues. I had developed a confidence in my movements that hadn't existed a year earlier. The human body was a fascinating and challenging medium, and I couldn't wait to practice more. Although we wear the same long white coat, I had no desire to be a butcher.

I had followed Dr. Organ's advice. I maintained my integrity. I tried to do the right thing. I'm far from perfect, but that's why residency is five years long.

*

I went to Lisa's wedding and nailed the sonnet. Right after the "O no!" I realized there was a bunch of people looking at me. My heart stopped for a second, but then it started again. I realized that they only wanted to hear me read the sonnet. Nobody wanted to lynch me, at least not until the wedding was over.

As I read and memorized the sonnet, I also analyzed it. And I agreed with it. True love wasn't halted by impediments. That was the premise of "Romeo and Juliet." If Rachel and I had true love, then the distance between us made no difference. That only left two possibilities. Either we made a big mistake, or we didn't have true love.

I opted for the former. I loved her. I tried to call her from the wedding that night to tell her, but she wasn't home.

At dinner, Lisa's father asked me if I was still dating the same girl he had met at our medical school graduation a year before.

I explained that I wasn't.

He told me, "Don't worry, when you're in practice, women will be breaking down your door."

I chortled. That moment was always being moved farther away. When I was in high school my mom had said that women would me beating down my door in college. When I started college I had heard, "Wait until you are in medical school, a guy like you...'" But then I was in medical school, and nobody had beaten down my door—I should know, I had studied right behind it for four years. Instead, I was told to wait until residency. "Now you're saying wait until I'm in practice," I told Lisa's dad. "Next it will be, 'Wait until you retire. Girls will be beating down your door to cart you around in your wheelchair.'"

He laughed.

But I wasn't joking.

Two days later, I finally got in touch with Rachel. I excitedly told her about what I had done the past few days. I told her that I called her the other day. Then she told me that she had gone out on two dates.

The words walloped me. I fell to the couch. "With the same guy?"

"Yes."

I didn't know what to say. What could I say?

"Do you want to talk about it?" she asked.

"I don't know what to say," I said. "I guess that was the reason we broke up."

"Yeah."

We sat in silence while thoughts raced through my head. I still loved her. We broke up a mere twenty-nine days ago. If she already went out with someone else then she wasn't as interested in me as I thought. What happened to not being able to imagine dating anyone else anytime soon? She said that if she dated someone else that it would likely be the person she married? Why hadn't she told me to sit down before telling me?

"Do you want to talk about this?" she asked again.

"I don't know what to say. I still love you."

"I love you, too."

Just not like you used to, I thought. "You could have told me to sit down first."

"Sorry, I just had to blurt it out. It was hard to tell you."

I tried to be glad that she did, but it didn't really work. We shared more moments of awkward silence and snippets of meaningless conversation. Then it was time to go. We said our good-byes and she didn't hang up right away. I waited.

"What are you doing?" I asked.

"Nothing."

"Hang up."

"No, I am waiting for you."

"No, you don't do that anymore."

"Since when?"

"Since you told me you were going to break up with me."

"Really?"

"Yes. You hung up first then and ever since."

"Well. I am waiting this time."

"Okay. Good-bye." I hung up. How do things like that end up meaning so much? It's just hanging up. Maybe that's what love was, assigning meaning to all the little things.

I called Rachel back a minute later to apologize for zinging her at the end of the conversation. What I had said about hanging up, although true, was not fair.

So, my romance with Rachel ended right along with my General Surgery internship.

*

And because nothing should ever end sadly, here's a joke:

What's the difference between a rectal thermometer and an oral thermometer?

The taste.

EPILOGUE

Life didn't stop when the intern year ended. Beetle left the program for anesthesiology. Over the course of the next year, Evan and another member of my class left. Kendra went into family practice. Brodie also switched into anesthesiology. Even the Intern of the Year, a woman I rarely saw, left G-surg for Ortho. Two other interns were dismissed. John left for a plastic surgery fellowship.

Corey began his practice. He has more than enough work and his patients are surviving. He told me he wanted to send Dr. Landa a letter thanking him for teaching him what not to do. His wife is pregnant again. I guess that's what happens if you spend time at home.

My life changed incredibly in the four weeks since my internship began.

The camaraderie among residents and attendings puts the previous year to shame. I am doing more operating than ever before and am learning at a phenomenal rate. I'm doing what I'll be doing for the rest of my life; picking noses! And the people harass me! It's about time I feel accepted.

And I take call from home. I was on call July Fourth and didn't go into the hospital once. Too bad I didn't have anyone to spend it with.

I miss Rachel. I saved a message from her on my answering machine just in case it is the last I ever hear from her.

And, despite being a big, smart doctor, I still can't believe people let me cut them, even if it is in a mutually beneficial manner.

I painted a new picture.

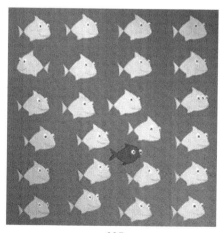

APPENDIX A

A picture of the appendix.

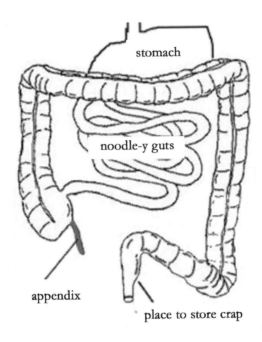

stomach

noodle-y guts

appendix

place to store crap

If you got this far, thanks for reading. If you enjoyed it, tell a friend about it (and leave a review on Amazon!). If you didn't, I really have to applaud your ability to stick through things. If you've found mistakes, let me know: sneakyelf@hotmail.com This book is self-published, so if you own a publishing company and have the irresistible urge to distribute this biography to the rest of the world, please contact me. It's a normal feeling.

For people who like "liking" things:
www.facebook.com/theyeartheytriedtokillme

I'll be putting additions to Chapter 27 on the Facebook page.

APPENDIX B

Tips to Becoming a Good Surgeon:

1. Never lie. Maintain your integrity. You cannot get it back.

2. Be compassionate. Every patient is seeing you because they are frightened that they need an operation. Never invalidate their fears/emotions with a simple "Don't worry." Give them the facts and let them calm themselves as they hear your confident explanation.

3. Be confident without being cocky. It can become a fine line when you are regarded as a lifesaver. A surgeon is no more special than a bus driver, the pope, or the guy who screws up your order at the drive-thru. But confidence is a necessity. People believe their life is in your hands. Your uncertainty will frighten them.

4. Become God-like. What better surgeon could there be than God? Omniscient and omnipotent. Every surgery is a miraculous success in the eyes of the patient. There's a saying: "If the patient lives, thank God. If the patient dies, blame the doctor." See, better to be God. Just remember rule 3, gods haven't been cocky since the Ancient Greeks.

5. Don't speak above patient's heads. Nine years of training leaves you with a vocabulary no one else understands. Learn how to speak in your patient's language without belittling them.

6. Be a surgeon without only being a surgeon. One-dimensional people are boring. The only reason to hang out with them is to make yourself appear more dynamic.

7. Work hard; work efficiently. This isn't a secret; it is a necessity. If you aren't working hard, at least look like you are! Otherwise, people will give you work to do. Brodie's disheveled hair fooled everyone.

8. Trust no one. Okay, I learned that one from the X-Files.

9. Do not let a patient dictate their plan of health. If a patient wants you to do something and it makes you uneasy, DON'T DO IT!

10. Do not become a dictator of your patient's health. Make them understand why you think your plan is necessary. Explain the more and less aggressive choices and let them choose. Most people want to feel like they are in control. If those tactics don't work, prescribe potent painkillers so they are too sauced to argue.

11. Don't be the hammer that only sees nails. You need to look at the whole problem.

12. Don't complain. Everyone thinks they are overworked, even some actors who get twenty million dollars a film.

13. Everything that can go wrong will go wrong at some time. This isn't quite Murphy's Law. You will see every possible error and outcome for every disease. Many of them you will never see again. Learn something from every failure to avoid repeating it. The real trick is not to become obsessive about avoiding error to the point that it impairs your abilities to function efficiently. In order to be a great surgeon, immediately after learning each lesson you must deny that it ever happened and when you are busted, blame it on the resident.

14. A fortune cookie fortune once told me, "If you fail to plan you plan to fail." For every surgery, have everything you might need available. And, if possible, always have an assistant, if only to be a gopher.

15. Always have your patient lie down in the fetal position to do a rectal exam. If you have them standing, leaning over the exam table you will find yourself in an awkward position when your nervous patient passes out. It isn't easy to hold someone upright with just your finger up their butt.

16. American culture dictates that the naked human body is embarrassing. Try to preserve your patient's dignity by explaining what you are going to do and then only undraping what is necessary for the exam. (Then laugh at them behind closed doors.)

17. Use plenty of anesthesia on awake patients; sedate them as much as possible. You don't want an uncomfortable patient kicking you during his colonoscopy and you definitely don't want him remembering he was in enough pain that he kicked you.

18. "Unthinking respect for authority is the greatest enemy of truth." That's a quote from Al Einstein. It's true. It is the mandatory quote the author finds important enough to share with his audience. A quote that, if alone on the front page, is supposed to inspire. I could not put it alone at the front of the book because I thought, "All right, stop, collaborate and listen…" would have been a more amusing way to start things off. But Vanilla Ice wouldn't give me permission.

19. Make friends with the nurses. If you write a book that shows mainly their bad sides, apologize. Being woken up repeatedly in the middle of the night is not an excuse to disparage the entire profession.

20. Lastly, if you must put strawberries in your vagina, please remember to count them on the way in and the way out.

ACKNOWLEDGMENTS

Thanks to everyone who encouraged me to write this adventure. Cohan Andersen was the first to recognize my diary, my catharsis, might actually be a story other people want to read...despite it not having zombies.

Thanks to Misty Urban for editing, encouraging, and helping me get two excerpts published. Thanks to David Hicks for helping edit it into a finished product and Kristen House for finding the (hopefully) last mistakes. My gratitude goes out to Tyler and Ange McQuade, Lisa Jewell, and my mom for all the tidbits and advice. A number of you read this in various stages and your feedback helped immensely.

Thanks to Zeppelin and Jinx for sitting at my feet, just waiting for a walk, while I revised for hours.

Last, but never least: Thanks to Vivian for being my cheerleader and the love of my life.

PS. Thanks to all the patients, doctors, nurses, techs, and scrub techs for teaching me.

ABOUT THE AUTHOR

Salvatore Iaquinta is a part-time author and full time surgeon in the San Francisco Bay Area. After spending years of his life looking for the ultimate joke, he discovered that the joke is life itself. He now lives by the motto "Laughter is the best medicine, but surgery is a close second." It's working; some of his patients will attest that his operative technique is laughable.

Alright, I can't talk about myself in the third-person.

I love making things. Anything. Whether it is creating a way to reconstruct a disfiguring wound, sewing a dog toy, or designing a puzzle, I am constantly making something. I wrote a daily comic strip for the University of Madison's "Badger Herald". I've had two excerpts of my book "The Year They Tried to Kill Me: Surviving a surgical internship even if the patient's don't" published. One of which, "What am I Doing Here?", won an award in a physician's writing contest.

My original goal for "The Year They Tried to Kill Me" was to tell people what it takes to become a surgeon. The gritty stories would scare students from becoming surgeons. But somewhere along the way I realized I just wanted to write a story to amuse people; a glimpse behind the scenes that lets them know their stoic doctor is actually human...a fallible human.

Enjoy!